Contemporary Diagnosis
and Management of

# The Patient With
# Type 2 Diabetes®

Barry J. Goldstein, MD, PhD, FACE, Editor
Professor of Medicine, Biochemistry, and
Molecular Pharmacology, and
Director, Division of Endocrinology,
Diabetes, and Metabolic Diseases
Jefferson Medical College of
Thomas Jefferson University
Philadelphia, PA
*and*

Jeffrey L. Miller, MD, FACP, FACE
Serge Jabbour, MD, FACP, FACE
Intekhab Ahmed, MD, FACP, FACE
Kevin Furlong, DO
Cheryl Marco, RD, CDE

*First Edition*

Published by Handbooks in Health Care Co.,
Newtown, Pennsylvania, USA

This book has been prepared and is presented as a service to the medical community. The information provided reflects the knowledge, experience, and personal opinions of Barry J. Goldstein, MD, PhD, Professor of Medicine, Biochemistry, and Molecular Pharmacology, and Director, Division of Endocrinology, Diabetes, and Metabolic Diseases, Jefferson Medical College of Thomas Jefferson University, Philadelphia, PA, as well as those of his colleagues in the Division of Endocrinology, Diabetes, and Metabolic Diseases: Intekhab Ahmed, MD, FACP, FACE, Associate Professor of Clinical Medicine; Serge Jabbour, MD, FACP, FACE, Associate Professor of Clinical Medicine; Jeffrey L. Miller, MD, FACP, FACE, Clinical Professor of Medicine; Kevin Furlong, DO, Assistant Professor of Clinical Medicine; Vanita Treat, MD, Fellow in Endocrinology, Thomas Jefferson University Hospital; and Cheryl Marco, RD, CDE, Coordinator, Diabetes Education and Weight Management Programs.

**This book is not intended to replace or to be used as a substitute for the complete prescribing information prepared by each manufacturer for each drug. Because of possible variations in drug indications, in dosage information, in newly described toxicities, in drug/drug interactions, and in other items of importance, reference to such complete prescribing information is definitely recommended before any of the drugs discussed are used or prescribed.**

International Standard Book Number: 978-1-931981-80-4

Library of Congress Catalog Card Number: 2007936283

# Table of Contents

# Chapter 1

# Pathophysiology of Hyperglycemia in Type 2 Diabetes

The practicing clinician will see an increasing number of type 2 diabetes cases in the United States because the condition is expanding in the adult population and extending into the younger population. The prevalence of type 2 diabetes in the United States has reached about 6% of the total population. One study recently showed that about 4% of obese white adolescents currently have diabetes and an additional 21% have abnormal glucose tolerance.[1] Most patients have the common form of type 2 diabetes, which has a multifactorial pathogenesis due to alterations in several gene products, exacerbated by overweight and sedentary lifestyles. Diabetes management is focused on comprehensive risk factor management, including glycemia, lipids, and hypertension, to prevent the devastating complications of diabetes, which usually involve the vascular consequences of accelerated atherogenesis.

## Insulin Resistance

Normal glucose metabolism requires a coordinated balance of hepatic glucose production (eg, glycogenolysis, gluconeogenesis) and glucose uptake into skeletal muscle and adipose tissue in fasting and postprandial states under the direction of a symphony of neural influences and circulating hormones, especially involving insulin, glucagon, and the incretins (Figure 1-1). The close association between

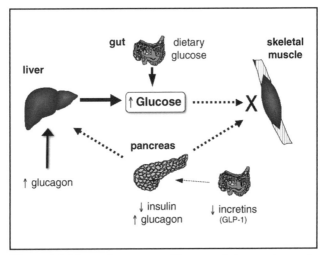

**Figure 1-1:** The major sources of increased plasma glucose in type 2 diabetes. The steady-state plasma-glucose concentration is determined by the balance of hepatic glucose output, disposal of glucose by skeletal muscle (a major site of glucose metabolism and storage), and absorption of dietary carbohydrates during meals. In type 2 diabetes, excessive hepatic glucose production and decreased muscle glucose uptake occur because of resistance to the action of circulating insulin and decreased β-cell insulin secretory capacity. The α-cells of the pancreatic islets are also dysfunctional and secrete excessive glucagon, which contribute to increased glucose output from the liver. Defects in the incretin system, primarily involving glucagon-like peptide-1 (GLP-1), also contribute to the secretion of defective insulin and glucagon from the pancreatic islets.

obesity and resistance to the biologic actions of insulin in glucose and lipid metabolism recognized for many years has provided insight into how adipose tissue also plays a major role in glucose regulation.[2] Intra-abdominal fat, in particular, has been associated with insulin resistance and abnormal glucose metabolism (ie, dysglycemia) as well as a set of pathogenic metabolic alterations (eg, hypertension, elevated triglycerides [Tgs], reduced high-density-lipoprotein cholesterol [HDL-C]), which comprise the cardiometabolic risk cluster (see Chapter 2). The visceral fat compartment influences insulin action through several physiologic mechanisms that are currently an active area of investigation (Figure 1-2).

Adipose tissue is now understood to be an active secretory organ; some of the secreted proteins that are specific products of adipose tissue have been designated as adipokines, and include leptin and adiponectin. In addition, adipose tissue releases a host of substances including metabolites such as free fatty acids (FFAs), cytokines (eg, tumor necrosis factor-$\alpha$ [TNF-$\alpha$]), signaling proteins (eg, angiotensin II [Ang II]), hormones, complement factors, and regulators of atherothrombosis (eg, plasminogen activator inhibitor-1 [PAI-1]).[3] Alterations in the circulating levels of these substances make important contributions to the insulin-resistant state characteristic of visceral obesity. In addition, they exert adverse effects in vascular endothelial and smooth muscle cells, effectively linking obesity and type 2 diabetes with endothelial dysfunction in the early inflammatory stages of atherosclerosis.[4] Indeed, the major long-term complication suffered by patients with type 2 diabetes is cardiovascular disease (CVD).

In obesity that occurs through continued overfeeding, the visceral adipocytes become resistant to the action of insulin, which normally suppresses the release of FFAs from stored Tgs.[5] The increase in circulating FFAs leads to higher levels of fatty acid molecules within skeletal muscle and liver cells, which contribute to insulin resistance in these tissues by the activation of signaling kinases, including protein kinase C, some isoforms of which oppose the insulin action cascade at the receptor tyrosine kinase and its tyrosine phosphorylated substrate proteins. FFAs may also induce skeletal muscle insulin resistance by activating the hexosamine pathway or by changing the fatty acid composition of membrane phospholipids, impairing mem-

7

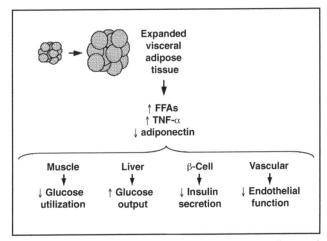

**Figure 1-2:** The effect of obesity on glucose metabolism and endothelial function is mediated by adipose tissue secretory products. With the expansion of the visceral adipose compartment, adipocytes release excessive amounts of several mediators, including FFAs and cytokines (ie, TNF-α). These substances contribute to insulin resistance in skeletal muscle and the liver, and adversely affect pancreatic insulin secretion and vascular endothelial function, which contributes to cardiovascular disease (CVD) risk in obesity and type 2 diabetes. In a complementary fashion, secretion of the protein adiponectin is decreased in obesity. However, since adiponectin exerts salutary effects, the reduction in circulating adiponectin causes a loss of its beneficial effects in skeletal muscle and liver insulin signaling as well as in endothelial function. FFAs=free fatty acids; TNF-α=tumor necrosis factor-α.

brane fluidity. Additional pathogenic signaling pathways that suppress insulin signaling are triggered by increased levels of cytokines (ie, TNF-α, interleukin-6 [IL-6]).

Adiponectin is unique in that the levels of this adipose-specific protein are reduced in both obesity and insulin-resistant states. Normally, adiponectin circulates in large oligomeric complexes at high concentrations in the bloodstream (2 to 10 μg/mL) where it exerts salutary effects on insulin signaling and has protective and anti-inflammatory effects in the vasculature.[6] In visceral obesity, adiponectin secretion may be impaired because the enlarged visceral adipocytes cannot efficiently assemble the adiponectin protein complexes.

Impaired mitochondrial function is a genetically determined component of the pathogenesis of type 2 diabetes that may also be exacerbated by changes in the circulating factors discussed above.[7] Defective mitochondrial lipid oxidation contributes to the accumulation of Tgs and other fatty acid derivatives in liver and skeletal muscle cells, which further impairs insulin signaling. Nonalcoholic steatohepatosis (ie, fatty liver) is a common clinical feature in insulin-resistant, obese patients that leads to transaminase elevation and can be recognized in an abdominal ultrasound.

## β-Cell Dysfunction

In response to the insulin resistance associated with visceral obesity, pancreatic β-cell insulin secretion is augmented to maintain glucose levels close to or within the normal range.[8] Consequently, most obese patients are insulin resistant, hyperinsulinemic, and frequently exhibit a range of glycemic abnormalities, including impaired fasting glucose (IFG) and impaired glucose tolerance (IGT) (ie, states of prediabetes). However, in about one third of overweight patients, the β-cell secretory impairment is sufficient enough to cause a rise in hyperglycemia to the level of diagnostic diabetes. A relative secretory inadequacy of the β-cell is, therefore, a fundamental cause of type 2 diabetes. Consistent with this pathophysiology, many of the genetic abnormalities found to be associated with type 2 diabetes regulate the development or function of pancreatic β-cells as well as the genes involved in insulin resistance.[9]

The development of clinically significant β-cell secretory failure is also associated with several abnormalities common to the obese state, including disrupted fat metabolism, hyperglycemia, and oxidative stress.[8] Although cellular FFAs are required as metabolic fuel for glucose-coupled insulin secretion, when chronically elevated, FFAs increase oxidative stress and impair signaling in β-cells. Hyperglycemia itself is a primary cause of β-cell inadequacy that has been defined as glucotoxicity. Even mild elevations of normal glucose levels may raise the set point of insulin secretion by mechanisms that are poorly understood. A key feature of the glucose-induced defect in insulin secretion is that it is specific for glucose, and other insulin secretion enhancers (eg, specific amino acids or sulfonylureas [glimepiride (Amaryl®), glyburide (DiaBeta®, Glynase®, Micronase®), glipizide (Glucotrol®, Glucotrol XL®)]) remain capable of stimulating insulin secretion. This effect may contribute to the clinical observation of fasting hyperglycemia with improved daytime glucose control. During the night, β-cell insulin secretion is stimulated only by excessive glucose released by the liver, and, if the β-cells experience glucotoxicity, they may not be able to manifest the level of insulin secretion that they can during the day, especially when a patient is taking daytime oral medications.

In insulin-resistant patients with hyperinsulinemia, β-cell hypersecretion of insulin also leads to excessive co-secretion of amylin, a β-cell hormone that aids in glucose regulation by suppressing glucagon, slowing gastric emptying, and suppressing appetite.[10] Amylin can be deposited in the pancreas as amyloid aggregates and also contributes to β-cell dysfunction. This dysfunction may help explain the clinical finding that sulfonylureas, which stimulate excessive insulin and amylin secretion in their mechanism of action to control glucose, fail more readily over time than other agents that reduce insulin secretion by enhancing the action of endogenous insulin (ie, thiazolidinediones [TZDs] [Actos® (pioglitazone), Avandia® (rosiglitazone), Avandamet® (rosiglitazone/metformin)], and metformin [Glucophage®, Glucophage® XR, Glumetza™, Riomet®]).

### *Dysregulated Glucagon Secretion*

Glucagon, a major counterregulatory hormone for insulin, plays a key role in glucose homeostasis. In the fasting state, as plasma-glucose and insulin levels fall, glucagon secretion from the β-cells of the pancreatic islets increases.[11] This increase in glucagon helps to modulate glucose production by the liver, effectively preventing fasting hypoglycemia. In the fed state, as rising plasma glucose stimulates insulin secretion, glucagon secretion is diminished, helping to reduce the postprandial rise in plasma glucose.

In type 2 diabetes, an imbalance in secretory dynamics develops between insulin and glucagon. Glucagon levels increase, leading to excessive hepatic glucose production and rising plasma-glucose levels. The suppression of glucagon levels that normally occurs during absorption of food is impaired, contributing to the sustained rise of plasma- glucose levels in hyperglycemic patients. Excessive glucagon secretion also contributes to elevated glucose levels that usally occur between meals and in the fasting state.

## Role of the Incretin System

Incretins (ie, glucagon-like peptide-1 [GLP-1], gastric inhibitory polypeptide [GIP]) are intestinal hormones that are released after eating, which play an important role in glucose homeostasis.[12] Physiologically, incretins enhance insulin release in a glucose-dependent manner, ie, insulin secretion is augmented by GLP-1 and GIP only when glucose levels are elevated, thus providing an effective barrier against hypoglycemia from these insulin secretion enhancers. GLP-1 also has the important effect of suppressing α-cell glucagon secretion in a glucose-dependent manner. GLP-1 also inhibits gastric emptying and reduces food intake and body weight. In contrast, GIP does not inhibit α-cell glucagon secretion, has minimal effect on gastric emptying, and has no significant effect on satiety or body weight.

Because the GLP-1 level is reduced in type 2 diabetes, but tissue responsiveness to GLP-1 is preserved, this pathway has emerged as an important therapeutic target. In contrast, GIP secretion is normal in patients with type 2 diabetes, but the response to GIP is muted, making the GIP receptor a poor target for therapeutic intervention.

## Summary

Insulin resistance and impaired β-cell insulin secretion are major pathophysiologic defects that lead to type 2 diabetes in susceptible people. Excessive visceral adipose tissue in obesity also contributes to these metabolic abnormalities. In addition, glucagon and the incretin system play a major role in the pathophysiology of hyperglycemia. These multiple defects are discussed more fully in later chapters as potential targets of available agents for the treatment of diabetes, providing a clear rationale for various combination therapies to effectively control plasma-glucose levels.

## References

1.    Sinha R, Fisch G, Teague B, et al: Prevalence of impaired glucose tolerance among children and adolescents with marked obesity. *N Engl J Med* 2002;346:802-810.

2.    Reaven G, Abbasi F, McLaughlin T: Obesity, insulin resistance, and cardiovascular disease. *Recent Prog Horm Res* 2004;59: 207-223.

3.    Kershaw EE, Flier JS: Adipose tissue as an endocrine organ. *J Clin Endocrinol Metab* 2004;89:2548-2556.

4.    Fantuzzi G, Mazzone T: Adipose tissue and atherosclerosis: exploring the connection. *Arterioscler Thromb Vasc Biol* 2007;27: 996-1003.

5.    Stumvoll M, Goldstein BJ, van Haeften TW: Type 2 diabetes: principles of pathogenesis and therapy. *Lancet* 2005;365:1333-1346.

6.    Goldstein BJ, Scalia R: Adipokines and vascular disease in diabetes. *Curr Diab Rep* 2007;7:25-33.

7.   Savage DB, Petersen KF, Shulman GI: Disordered lipid metabolism and the pathogenesis of insulin resistance. *Physiol Rev* 2007;87:507-520.

8.   Kahn SE: Clinical review 135: The importance of beta-cell failure in the development and progression of type 2 diabetes. *J Clin Endocrinol Metab* 2001;86:4047-4058.

9.   Sladek R, Rocheleau G, Rung J, et al: A genome-wide association study identifies novel risk loci for type 2 diabetes. *Nature* 2007;445:881-885.

10.  Riddle MC, Drucker DJ: Emerging therapies mimicking the effects of amylin and glucagon-like peptide 1. *Diabetes Care* 2006;29:435-449.

11.  Dunning BE, Gerich JE: The role of alpha-cell dysregulation in fasting and postprandial hyperglycemia in type 2 diabetes and therapeutic implications. *Endocr Rev* 2007;28:253-258.

12.  Drucker DJ: The biology of incretin hormones. *Cell Metabol* 2006;3:153-165.

# Chapter 2

# Insulin Resistance, Type 2 Diabetes, and the Cardiometabolic Syndrome

Type 2 diabetes develops from the interplay between increasing insulin resistance in skeletal muscle and liver, increasing hepatic glucose output, and decreasing insulin secretion caused by progressive pancreatic β-cell dysfunction as the result of lipotoxicity, glucose toxicity, and other factors. Type 2 diabetes develops in stages that correspond to the relative predominance of each of these physiologic factors as they relate to defects in insulin-mediated glucose uptake in skeletal muscle.

In the earliest stage of type 2 diabetes, insulin resistance is associated with hyperinsulinemia and, in general, excess visceral adiposity. The production of adipokines by adipose tissue is increasingly recognized as one important mediator of this relationship. Substances produced by fat, such as free fatty acids (FFAs), tumor necrosis factor-α (TNF-α), and leptin, suppress insulin-mediated glucose uptake. The greater the visceral adiposity, the higher the circulating levels of adipose-derived products. Genetic and environmental factors interact to determine adiposity and insulin resistance, as well as β-cell insulin secretion. With increasing age, components of the metabolic syndrome appear, defined by the National Cholesterol Education Program (NCEP) as the presence of three of the following five criteria:

- Fasting plasma glucose (FPG) >100 mg/dL
- Serum triglyceride (Tg) >150 mg/dL

- Serum high-density lipoprotein (HDL) <40 mg/dL
- Blood pressure >130/85 mm Hg
- Waist circumference >102 cm (40 inches) for men and >94 cm (37 inches) for women

Twenty to thirty percent of the US population has the metabolic syndrome.[1] In the next stage in the development of diabetes, pancreatic insulin production cannot keep up with insulin resistance in skeletal muscle and liver, resulting in a transition from normal glucose tolerance (NGT) to impaired glucose tolerance (IGT).[2] This stage is characterized by postprandial hyperglycemia (140 to 199 mg/dL), which is also associated with fasting hyperglycemia (100 to 125 mg/dL), although postprandial plasma glucose (PPG) is a more sensitive index of IGT. Because glucose uptake into muscle requires three to four times the amount of insulin needed to inhibit glucose production by the liver, in this stage, enough insulin is secreted to suppress hepatic glucose output and prevent the fasting plasma glucose (FPG) concentration from surpassing normal levels. However, as hepatic insulin resistance worsens, the liver begins to produce glucose in increasing amounts, which leads to the gradual increase in FPG that results in impaired fasting glucose (IFG).[3]

## Insulin Resistance, Type 2 Diabetes, and Risk of Cardiovascular Complications

Coronary artery disease (CAD) one of the life-threatening consequences of atherosclerosis, is the most common vascular complication of insulin resistance.[4] The age-adjusted prevalence of CAD in Americans with type 2 diabetes is two to four times of that in nondiabetic patients.[5] The manifestations of CAD, including angina pectoris, myocardial infarction (MI), and sudden death, are at least twice as common in patients with type 2 diabetes as in nondiabetic patients,[6] and, in certain studies, the incidence of these manifestations was nearly six times more common. For instance, in a large Finnish population study, the 7-year incidence of initial MI or death was 20% for patients with type 2 diabetes vs only 3.5% for nondiabetic patients.[7] This incidence for patients with diabetes was identical to that of nondiabetic subjects with known cardiovascular disease (CVD). As a result, the NCEP Adult Treatment Panel III (ATP III) considers diabetes as an atherosclerosis risk equivalent.[8] In the prospective Finnish study, patients with diabetes and known heart disease had a 45% incidence of recurrent MI.[9] The presence of severe CAD in diabetic patients results from the early development of atherosclerosis.[10] Accelerated atherogenesis and increased risk of CAD (generally twofold) are commonly found in prediabetic patients.[11] Patients with the metabolic syndrome as defined by the ATP III or World Health Organization (WHO) also have a substantially increased risk of CVD and mortality, as well as increased all-cause mortality.[12]

## Insulin Resistance Confers a Strong Risk of Type 2 Diabetes

The association between IGT and risk of developing type 2 diabetes has been documented in a wide range of racial and ethnic populations. In the San Antonio Heart Study (SAHS), the relative risk (RR) of developing type 2 diabetes conferred by IGT ranged from 4.3 to 7 depending upon race and sex.[7] By some estimates, as many as half of all individuals with IGT will develop type 2 diabetes after 10 years of follow-up, and this rate is considerably higher in groups with a high prevalence of diabetes.[5] Patients with IFG also have increased rates of late development of diabetes. Women with a history of gestational type 2 diabetes have the highest incidence of developing type 2 diabetes later in life (ie, 50% over 10 years). These patients need lifestyle recommendations as well as lifelong follow-up to prevent diabetes. Diabetes prevention is discussed in Chapter 3.

# References

1. Ford ES, Giles WH, Dietz WH: Prevalence of the metabolic syndrome among US adults: findings from the third National Health and Nutrition Examination Survey. *JAMA* 2002;287:356-359.

2. Nijpels G: Determinants for the progression from impaired glucose tolerance to non-insulin-dependent diabetes mellitus. *Eur J Clin Invest* 1998;29(suppl 2):8-13.

3. Reasner CA, Defronzo RA: Treatment of type 2 diabetes mellitus: a rational approach based on its pathophysiology. *Am Fam Physician* 2001;63:1687-1688.

4. Resnick HE, Howard BV: Diabetes and cardiovascular disease. *Annu Rev Med* 2002;52:245-267.

5. Gaede P, Vedel P, Larsen N, et al: Multifactorial intervention and cardiovascular disease in patients with type 2 diabetes. *N Engl J Med* 2003;348:383-393.

6. Laakso M: Cardiovascular disease in type 2 diabetes: challenge for treatment and prevention. *J Intern Med* 2001;249:225-235.

7. Beckman JA, Creager MA, Libby P: Diabetes and atherosclerosis: epidemiology, pathophysiology, and management. *JAMA* 2002;287:2570-2581.

8. Expert Panel on Detection, Evaluation, and Treatment of High Blood Cholesterol in Adults: Executive Summary of The Third Report of The National Cholesterol Education Program (NCEP) Expert Panel on Detection, Evaluation, And Treatment of High Blood Cholesterol In Adults (Adult Treatment Panel III). *JAMA* 2001;285:2486-2497.

9. Haffner SM: Coronary heart disease in patients with diabetes. *N Engl J Med* 2000;342:1040-1042.

10. Solomon CG: Reducing cardiovascular risk in type 2 diabetes. *N Engl J Med* 2003;348:457-459.

11. Galassi A, Reynolds K, He J: Metabolic syndrome and risk of cardiovascular disease: a meta-analysis. *Am J Med* 2006;119:812-819.

12. Hu FB, Stampfer MJ, Haffner SM: Elevated risk of cardiovascular disease prior to clinical diagnosis of type 2 diabetes. *Diabetes Care* 2002;25:1129-1134.

*Chapter* **3**

# Preventing Type 2 Diabetes

## Epidemiology

Type 2 diabetes is a worldwide pandemic associated with significant morbidity and mortality. The incidence of diabetes in the United States has increased by a monumental 61% between 1990 and 2001 and is believed to be related to both genetic and environmental factors (ie, too many calories of the wrong type and too little caloric expenditure).[1] Type 2 diabetes now affects about 5% of adults worldwide, and its prevalence is rapidly rising, causing a significant financial and public health burden on society.[2] Worldwide, the number of people affected with diabetes is projected to increase from 150 million today to 220 million by 2010 and 300 million by 2025.[2]

This chapter focuses on the early detection of who is most at risk for the development of type 2 diabetes and discusses possible early intervention strategies to prevent the progression to full-fledged diabetes and its numerous associated complications.

## Impaired Glucose Tolerance and Impaired Fasting Glucose

Those individuals who are on track to develop type 2 diabetes pass through a phase of impaired glucose tolerance (IGT).[3] β-Cell response plays a key role in the development of adult-onset diabetes. IGT does not pose a threat as long as pancreatic β-cells compensate for the increase in demand placed upon them by the state of insulin resistance. When β-cells fail to rise to this challenge, a state of glucose toxicity occurs, but this toxicity is potentially reversible with targeted lifestyle therapy (ie, diet, weight loss) or pharmacotherapy.

IGT is a phenomenon in the fed state that is between normal glucose tolerance (NGT) and full-fledged diabetes.[4] NGT is defined as fasting plasma glucose (FPG) <100 mg/dL and a 2-hour post-oral glucose tolerance test (OGTT) glucose value of <140 mg/dL. IGT is defined as a plasma-glucose concentration between 140 and 200 mg/dL after a 75 g glucose load in a patient with a FPG of <126 mg/dL. Impaired fasting glucose (IFG) is defined as a FPG concentration between 100 and 126 mg/dL.[6] IGT and IFG can overlap, but they can also occur in isolation as mutually exclusive entities. The prevalence of these conditions varies with race, sex, and age. Both IGT and IFG are associated with increased abdominal obesity, hyperinsulinemia, hypertension, elevated triglyceride (Tg) levels, and low high-density lipoprotein (HDL) levels, which are all significant risk factors for cardiovascular disease (CVD).[5]

More than 8% of adults worldwide suffer from either IGT or IFG or a combination of both conditions. Patients with high-risk prediabetic conditions have about a 25% to 50% lifetime risk of developing type 2 diabetes and should be targeted for primary intervention.[3]

## Clinical Trials

### The Finnish Diabetes Prevention Study

The Finnish Diabetes Prevention Study (FDPS) established a precedent for effectively altering lifestyle after the development of diabetes in high-risk patients with IGT.[6] Patients with IGT were randomized to a control group or a lifestyle intervention group with diet and exercise counseling. Average weight loss in the diet and exercise group reached 3.5 kg at 2 years, and, at 4 years, there was a much lower incidence of developing type 2 diabetes. The

**Table 3-1: A Summary of the Major Clinical Trials for the Prevention of Diabetes in Patients With Impaired Glucose Tolerance**

**Study**

Finnish Diabetes Prevention Study (FDPS) Group

Da Qing study

Diabetes Prevention Program (DPP) Research Group

Diabetes Reduction Assessment with Ramipril and Rosiglitazone Medication (DREAM) trial

Study to Prevent Noninsulin-dependent Diabetes Mellitus (STOP-NIDDM) trial

Acarbose (Precose®)
Metformin (Glucophage®, Glucophage® XR, Glumetza™, Riomet®)
Ramipril (Altace®)
Rosiglitazone (Avandia®)

lifestyle modification group showed a 58% relative risk (RR) reduction in the development of diabetes compared with the control group (Table 3-1), and continued effects were seen during the 3-year follow-up period (36% RR as a result of lifestyle change).

### The Da Qing Study

In China, the Da Qing study randomized 577 subjects with IGT to a control group or to one of three lifestyle alterations, which were diet control, exercise intervention,

| Therapy | Relative Risk Reduction |
|---|---|
| Diet + Exercise | 58% |
| | |
| Diet | 31% |
| Exercise | 46% |
| Diet + Exercise | 42% |
| | |
| Diet + Exercise | 58% |
| Metformin | 31% |
| | |
| Rosiglitazone + Diet + Exercise | 60% |
| | |
| Acarbose | 25% |

or a combination of diet and exercise.[7] In all three intervention groups, patients were found to have a reduction in the development of type 2 diabetes by 31% to 46% compared with the control group.

### The Diabetes Prevention Program

In the United States, the Diabetes Prevention Program (DPP) trial, a randomized, prospective clinical study, focused on the prevention of type 2 diabetes in high-risk patient populations (ie, those with IGT and/or IFG).[8]

The results of this study echoed the findings of the FDPS. The DPP was designed to determine the effect of modifying reversible risk factors through lifestyle changes or with the administration of metformin (Glucophage®, Glucophage® XR, Glumetza™, Riomet®) on the development of diabetes. Diabetes was the primary outcome as defined by the 1997 criteria of the American Diabetes Association (ADA), which was a FPG concentration of $\geq 126$ mg/dL or a plasma-glucose level of $\geq 200$ mg/dL 2 hours after the administration of a 75 g glucose load. The 3,234 prediabetic patients, followed for 2.8 years on average, were randomly assigned to receive a placebo, metformin (850 mg twice daily), or lifestyle modifications designed to induce at least a 7% weight loss and to include at least 150 minutes of exercise weekly. Both lifestyle intervention (58% RR reduction) and metformin (31% RR reduction) slowed the progression to diabetes in these high-risk patients. Intensive lifestyle modifications also resulted in the decrease of cardiovascular risk factors including hypertension, elevated Tgs, low HDL levels, and small dense low-density lipoprotein (LDL) levels.[5] If instituted in a timely fashion, these initial aggressive measures should allow for the delay and possibly the prevention of many complications of diabetes that comprise a large part of the public health burden of diabetes today.

## The TRIPOD Trial

The efficacy of thiazolidinediones (TZDs) in the treatment of type 2 diabetes was first seen during the Troglitazone in Prevention of Diabetes (TRIPOD) trial.[9] TZDs reduce insulin resistance and possibly preserve pancreatic β-cell function by improving glucose utilization by peripheral tissues, reducing hepatic glucose production, and promoting insulin secretion. In the TRIPOD trial, 266 Hispanic women with a history of gestational type 2 diabetes were randomized to 400 mg of troglitazone or placebo daily. There was a 5.4% incidence in diabetes yearly in the troglitazone group, compared with 12.1% incidence in the placebo group. Troglitazone, which was removed from the US market for liver safety concerns, was not the last of the TZDs to be studied for the prevention of diabetes.

### The DREAM Trial

Positive results of pharmacologic therapy with ramipril (Altace®) and rosiglitazone (Avandia®) have been the focus of the Diabetes Reduction Assessment with Ramipril and Rosiglitazone Medication (DREAM) trial.[10] The DREAM trial studied 5,269 adults who were at least 30 years of age with documented IFG, IGT, or both, without any prior known CVD. They were randomly assigned to receive either rosiglitazone (8 mg/day) or placebo and were followed for a median of 3 years. The DREAM study results suggest that rosiglitazone, used at 8 mg daily for 3 years and in combination with lifestyle recommendations, decreased the risk of type 2 diabetes or death by 60% and increased the return to normoglycemia (by 70% to 80% compared with placebo) in adults with IFG, IGT, or both. Beneficial effects on blood pressure were also found in those patients receiving rosiglitazone. There were 14 cases of nonfatal heart failure, representing 0.5% of subjects, in the rosiglitazone group compared with 2 (0.1%) in the placebo group, which warrants close observation. There were no differences in mortality between the rosiglitazone and placebo groups. Treatment with ramipril did not significantly lower the incidence of diabetes; however, it did result in an improved glucose profile after a glucose load. Despite promising findings from this study, careful further study is required to determine the true benefits of such drugs and whether their rewards really outweigh their risks in this patient population.

### The STOP-NIDDM Trial

Acarbose (Precose®), an α-glucosidase inhibitor, lowers postprandial plasma glucose (PPG) levels and reduces β-cell demand. The Study to Prevent Noninsulin-dependent Diabetes Mellitus (STOP-NIDDM) trial was a double-blind, placebo-controlled trial that randomized patients with IGT to either 100 mg of acarbose or placebo three times daily.[11] The primary end point of the study was the development of diabetes as determined by a yearly OGTT. Of the 682 patients in the acarbose group, 32% developed diabetes, compared with 42% of the 686 patients in the placebo group. The risk of developing type 2 diabetes over 3.3 years in the patients with IGT was decreased by 25%. Common side effects of acarbose included flatulence and diarrhea. This study, like the DPP, reminds us that pharmacologic intervention in addition to lifestyle change plays an important role in the spectrum of plasma-glucose control.

CVD accounts for 60% to 70% of deaths in patients with type 2 diabetes, and the reduction of this death rate is an important objective in the analysis of the influence of pharmacologic agents like acarbose. The STOP-NIDDM trial, the first prospective intervention study to look at the effect of diabetes prevention on CVD, showed a 49% RR reduction in the development of cardiovascular events (especially myocardial infarction [MI]) as a result of lowering postprandial hyperglycemia.[12] Acarbose also resulted in a 34% RR reduction in new cases of hypertension and a 5.3% absolute risk reduction in its incidence.[12] Because CVD is prevalent among both diabetics and those with IGT, the positive effects of acarbose on CVD risk factors are of substantial value.

## Conclusions

Lifestyle modifications (ie, diet, exercise) prevailed by lowering the incidence of diabetes by >50% over pharmacologic therapy, as suggested by the numerous clinical trials above, although many medications show promise in reducing the incidence of diabetes and decreasing the risk factors associated with CVD when used correctly and monitored closely. It appears that those with the highest risk (ie, those with IGT, IFG, or both), would be the most likely to benefit from early preventive strategies. These individuals should receive appropriate counseling in diet and nutrition, weight-loss strategies, and individualized exercise programs. Based upon the aforementioned clinical trials, preventive medications should be considered when appropriate and discussed with each patient on an individual basis.

A consensus statement was issued by the ADA about how to treat those patients with IGT and/or IFG. After review of the data published by the aforementioned studies, the following considerations for the treatment of IGT and IFG were recommended by the ADA:

- For individuals with IFG or IGT, lifestyle modification, 5% to 10% weight loss, and 30 min/day of moderate physical activity is suggested.[5]
- For individuals with IFG and IGT, and any of the following—age <60, body mass index (BMI) >35 kg/m$^2$, family history of diabetes in first-degree relatives, high Tgs, low HDL-C level, hypertension, or glycosylated hemoglobin $A_{1c}$ (Hb$A_{1c}$) >6%—lifestyle change and/or initiation of metformin is recommended.[5]

## References

1. Mokdad AH, Ford ES, Bowman BA, et al: Prevalence of obesity, diabetes and obesity-related health risk factors, 2001. *JAMA* 2003;289:76-79.

2. Zimmet P, Alberti KG, Shaw J: Global and societal implications of the diabetes epidemic. *Nature* 2001;414:782-787.

3. Nathan DM, Davidson MB, DeFronzo RA, et al, and the American Diabetes Association: Impaired fasting glucose and impaired glucose tolerance. *Diabetes Care* 2007;30:753-759.

4. Genuth S, Alberti KG, Bennett P, et al, and the Expert Committee on the Diagnosis and Classification of Diabetes Mellitus: Follow-up report on the diagnosis of diabetes mellitus. *Diabetes Care* 2003;26:3160-3167.

5.   Ratner R, Goldberg R, Haffner S, et al, and the Diabetes Prevention Program Research Group: Impact of intensive lifestyle and metformin therapy on cardiovascular disease risk factors in the diabetes prevention program. *Diabetes Care* 2005;28:888-894.

6.   Tuomilehto J, Lindstrom J, Eriksson JG, et al, and the Finnish Diabetes Prevention Study group: Prevention of type 2 diabetes mellitus by changes in lifestyle among subjects with impaired glucose tolerance. *N Engl J Med* 2001;344:1343-1350.

7.   Pan XR, Li GW, Hu YH, et al: Effects of diet and exercise in preventing NIDDM in people with impaired glucose tolerance. The Da Qing IGT and Diabetes Study. *Diabetes Care* 1997;20:537-544.

8.   Knowler WC, Barrett-Conner E, Fowler SE, et al, and the Diabetes Prevention Program Research Group: Reduction in the incidence of type 2 diabetes with lifestyle intervention or metformin. *N Engl J Med* 2002;346:393-403.

9.   Buchanan TA, Xiang AH, Peters RK, et al: Preservation of pancreatic beta-cell function and prevention of type 2 diabetes by pharmacological treatment of insulin resistance in high-risk hispanic women. *Diabetes* 2002;51:2796-2803.

10.   Gerstein HC, Yusuf S, Bosch J, et al, and the DREAM (Diabetes Reduction Assessment withy Ramipril and Rosiglitazone Medication) Trial Investigators: Effect of rosiglitazone on the frequency of diabetes in patients with impaired glucose tolerance or impaired fasting glucose: a randomised controlled trial. *Lancet* 2006;368:1096-1105; erratum *Lancet* 2006;368:1770.

11.   Chiasson JL, Josse RG, Gomis R, et al, and the STOP-NIDDM Trial Research Group: Acarbose for prevention of type 2 diabetes mellitus: the STOP-NIDDM randomised trial. *Lancet* 2002;359:2072-2077.

12.   Chiasson JL, Josse RG, Gomis R, et al, and the STOP-NIDDM Trial Research Group: Acarbose treatment and the risk of cardiovascular disease and hypertension in patients with impaired glucose tolerance: the STOP-NIDDM trial. *JAMA* 2003;290:486-494.

# Chapter 4

# Rationale for Glucose Control and Goals of Therapy

T he primary treatment goal in diabetes is to prevent both acute and chronic complications. To accomplish this goal, one has to keep in mind that diabetes is a multisystemic disease. It often exists in the presence of other comorbidities that work synergistically with hyperglycemia to produce its dreaded complications, which is why the goals of therapy established by the American Diabetes Association (ADA) and the American Association of Clinical Endocrinologists (AACE) focus not only on glycemic control, but also on blood-pressure control, lipid control, and risk factor modification. In fact, it has been shown that long-term, intensified intervention aimed at multiple risk factors in patients with type 2 diabetes and microalbuminuria reduces the risk of cardiovascular and microvascular events by about 50%.[1] In this chapter, we will review the goals of therapy in diabetes management and provide support for their existence. The specific strategies to achieve these goals will be addressed in later chapters.

## Glycemia

Glycemic control is a fundamental goal in the management of diabetes. A number of trials have demonstrated the importance of glycemic control in preventing microvascular and macrovascular complications. The ADA and

## Table 4-1: ADA Goals for Glycemic Control

| | |
|---|---|
| Hemoglobin $A_{1c}$ ($HbA_{1c}$) | <7% |
| Preprandial plasma-glucose level | 90 to 130 mg/dL |
| Peak postprandial plasma glucose (PPG) level | <180 mg/dL |

ADA=American Diabetes Association

## Table 4-2: ACE Goals for Glycemic Control

| | |
|---|---|
| Hemoglobin $A_{1c}$ ($HbA_{1c}$) | <6.5% |
| Preprandial plasma-glucose level | <110 mg/dL |
| 2-hour postprandial plasma glucose (PPG) level | <140 mg/dL |

ACE=American College of Endocrinology

the American College of Endocrinology (ACE) have established general glycemic targets as shown in Tables 4-1 and 4-2.[2,3] However, most experts agree that the glycemic goal in any individual patient is normoglycemia. This goal is not based on any randomized prospective trials but on epidemiologic data that shows no lower limit of glycosylated hemoglobin $A_{1c}$ ($HbA_{1c}$) at which further lowering does not reduce the risk of complications.[4] However, there are exceptions to this goal. Tight glycemic control may not be desirable in patients who have limited life expectancies, a history of repeated hypoglycemia, are very young children, are elderly, or in individuals with comorbid conditions.[2] Table 4-3 shows some of the key trials supporting the goal of glycemic control.[4-7]

## Inpatient Setting

A disproportionate number of hospitalized patients has type 2 diabetes, and this number is increasing. Multiple studies have shown that inpatient hyperglycemia is associated with increased morbidity and mortality in diabetic and nondiabetic patients, and an increasing number of trials are showing the beneficial effects of tighter glycemic control. Targets for inpatient glycemic control have been developed and promulgated by the ACE and the AACE (Table 4-4).[8] It is important to remember that these targets are only glycemic targets and should be individualized based on the specific clinical situation.

Data supporting the glycemic goals for not critically ill medical or surgical hospitalized patients are derived primarily from observational and retrospective studies. A retrospective review by Umpierrez et al[9] found a 2.5-fold increase in mortality in diabetic patients and an 18-fold increase in mortality in patients with hyperglycemia without a prior diagnosis of diabetes when compared with normoglycemic control subjects. Pomposelli et al[10] found that postoperative hyperglycemia is a sensitive predictor of nosocomial infection.

In patients with acute myocardial infarction (MI), hyperglycemia is a predictor of mortality in patients with and without diabetes.[11] The Diabetes and Insulin-Glucose Infusion in Acute Myocardial Infarction (DIGAMI) study randomized patients with acute MI to intravenous (IV) insulin with intensive insulin management or conventional therapy. In comparison with conventional therapy, intensive insulin therapy resulted in a 29% reduction in mortality at 1 year and a 28% reduction at 3.4 years.[12]

Trials have also shown that good glycemic control in patients undergoing cardiac surgery results in improved outcomes. Furnary et al[13,14] showed a 57% reduction in deep sternal wound infections and a 66% reduction in mortality in cardiac surgical patients who received a continuous IV insulin infusion compared with a historical control group

## Table 4-3: Major Studies to Support Glycemic Goals

| Trial | Description | HbA$_{1c}$ |
|-------|-------------|-----------|
| DCCT[4] | Prospective randomized trial of patients with type 2 diabetes | Intensive 7.2% Conventional 9.1% |
| DCCT/ EDIC[5] | Extension of DCCT study—93% of original DCCT participants were followed from study completion in 1993 until 2005. | Intensive 8.1% Conventional 8.1% |
| UKPDS[6] | Prospective randomized, observational study of patients with type 2 diabetes | Intensive 7% Conventional 7.9% |
| Kumamoto[7] | Prospective randomized trial of patients with type 2 diabetes | Intensive 7.2% Conventional 9.4% |

DCCT=Diabetes Control and Complications Trial; DCCT/EDIC=Diabetes Control and Complications Trial/Epidemiology of Diabetes Interventions and Complications Trial; HbA$_{1c}$=hemoglobin A$_{1c}$;UKPDS=United Kingdom Prospective Diabetes Study

## Results

Intensive insulin therapy reduced the adjusted mean risk for the development of diabetic retinopathy by 76%, slowed the progression of retinopathy by 54%, and reduced the development of proliferative or severe nonproliferative retinopathy by 47%. Intensive insulin therapy also reduced the occurrence of microalbuminuria by 39%, albuminuria by 54%, and clinical neuropathy by 60%. The chief adverse event associated with intensive insulin therapy was a two- to threefold increase in severe hypoglycemia.

Intensive insulin treatment reduced the risk of any cardiovascular disease (CVD) event by 42% and the risk of nonfatal myocardial infarction (MI), stroke, or death from CVD by 57%.

Each 1% reduction in updated mean glycosylated hemoglobin $A_{1c}$ (HbA$_{1c}$) was associated in reductions in risk of 21% for any end point related to diabetes, 21% for deaths related to diabetes, 14% for MI, and 37% for microvascular complications. No threshold was observed for any end point.

Intensive insulin therapy associated with a 68% relative risk (RR) reduction in sustained diabetic retinopathy and a 74% RR reduction in the development of microalbuminuria.

## Table 4-4: Inpatient Glycemic Targets

| Setting | Upper Limits for Glycemic Targets | |
| --- | --- | --- |
| | Premeal | Maximal plasma glucose |
| — | | |
| ICU | 80 to 110 mg/dL | 80 to110 mg/dL |
| Med/Surg | 110 mg/dL | <180 mg/dL |

ICU=intensive care unit; Med/Surg=general medical/surgical floors

that received intermittent subcutaneous insulin injections. Lazar et al[15] also showed a lower incidence of wound infection, atrial fibrillation, recurrent ischemia, and a shorter hospital stay in patients randomized to IV insulin infusion compared with patients randomized to subcutaneous insulin injections with a more liberalized glycemic goal.

Data to support targets for intensive care unit (ICU) patients are derived primarily from two prospective randomized trials. Van den Berghe et al[16] performed a randomized trial in a primarily surgical ICU in which intensive insulin therapy with a goal glucose level of 80 to 110 mg/dL was compared with conventional therapy. They were able to show a reduction in mortality rate by 34%, sepsis by 46%, renal failure necessitating dialysis by 41%, need for blood transfusion by 50%, and critical illness related to polyneuropathy by 44%. A subsequent trial by the same group performed with the same intensive glycemic goals in a medical intensive care unit (MICU) showed improvements in several ICU-related morbidities, such as renal dysfunction and prolonged mechanical ventilation. Interestingly, among the 433 patients who were in the MICU for <3 days, there was an increased mortality rate in the intensively treated group compared with those patients who received conventional therapy. However, after adjustments for baseline characteristics, this difference was not statistically significant.[17]

Other studies also support glycemic control but lead to questions about the optimal upper limit of glycemia. Krinsley et al[18] compared 800 patients admitted to an ICU or a MICU before the institution of an intensive glucose management protocol (mean plasma-glucose level=152.3 mg/dL) and 800 patients admitted after the protocol was in place (mean plasma-glucose level=130.7 mg/dL). The plasma-glucose level goal with the intensive insulin protocol was <140 mg/dL. When compared with conventional therapy, the intensive insulin therapy decreased hospital mortality by 29.3%, length of stay in the ICU or the MICU by 10.8%, new acute renal insufficiency by 75%, and the number of patients undergoing blood transfusions by 18.7%.[18] This glycemic threshold is higher than in the van den Berghe trials,[16,17] yet still showed improvement in morbidity and mortality with lower rates of hypoglycemia.

## Pregnancy

About 8% of all pregnancies in the United States are complicated by hyperglycemia.[19] Hyperglycemia exists either in the context of pre-existing type 1 diabetes or gestational type 2 diabetes. During the first trimester of pregnancy, hyperglycemia increases the risk of spontaneous abortion and fetal malformation. Later in pregnancy, it increases the risk of microsomia and metabolic complications at birth. Several studies have shown that tighter glycemic control during preconception, pregnancy, and labor and delivery can prevent these complications. According to AACE guidelines, the patient should ideally have a $HbA_{1c}$ <6%, fasting plasma glucose (FPG) level between 60 and 90 mg/dL, and 1-hour postprandial plasma glucose (PPG) level <120 mg/dL. During labor and delivery, plasma-glucose concentration should be maintained between 70 and 90 mg/dL.[3] The ADA is more liberal in that their goals are a FPG level of <95 mg/dL, a 1-hour PPG level <140 mg/dL, and a 2-hour PPG level <120 mg/dL. Regardless of which guidelines are followed, blood pressure should be maintained at <130/80 mm Hg.[2]

## Blood Pressure

Approximately 73% of patients with type 2 diabetes use prescription medications for hypertension or have a blood pressure ≥130/80 mm Hg.[20] This is significant because hypertension contributes to the development and progression of all vascular complications of diabetes, including renal disease, coronary artery disease (CAD), stroke, peripheral vascular disease (PVD), lower extremity amputations, and diabetic retinopathy. Clinical trials have demonstrated a linear relationship between blood pressure and diabetic nephropathy, and adverse cardiovascular events and mortality. In fact, hypertension may be a more significant risk factor for macrovascular complications than hyperglycemia itself.

The Seventh Report of the Joint National Committee on Prevention, Detection, Evaluation, and Treatment of High Blood Pressure (JNC 7), the National Kidney Foundation (NKF), ADA, ACE, and AACE all concur that the target blood pressure in patients with diabetes is <130/80 mg/dL. The literature also contains abundant data from large randomized, controlled trials to support this goal. In general, for every 10 mm Hg reduction in systolic blood pressure, the risk for any complication related to diabetes is reduced by 12%. Furthermore, blood pressure control reduces the risk of CVD by 33% to 50% and the risk of microvascular complications by about 33% in patients with diabetes.[20]

## Lipids

Diabetes accelerates the progression of atherosclerosis, coronary events, strokes, and peripheral arterial disease (PAD), and is, therefore, considered a cardiovascular risk

## Table 4-5: Lipoprotein Goals for Adults With Type 2 Diabetes

| Risk | LDL-C* | HDL-C | Triglycerides | Non-HDL Cholesterol |
|------|--------|-------|---------------|---------------------|
| Regular | <100 | >40 | <150 | <130 |
| High | <70 | >40 | <150 | <100 |

Data are given in mg/dL.

*ADA recommends that all type 2 diabetes patients over age 40 should be prescribed a statin to reduce their LDL-C by >30% to 40% regardless of baseline LDL.

HDL-C=high-density lipoprotein cholesterol; LDL-C=low-density lipoprotein cholesterol

equivalent. Cardiovascular events are two to four times more likely to occur in diabetic patients compared with nondiabetic patients and account for approximately 65% of deaths in this population.[20] The characteristic dyslipidemia in diabetes includes high low-density lipoprotein (LDL), more atherogenic small dense LDL, low high-density lipoprotein (HDL), and high Tgs.

Studies in diabetic patients have shown clear reductions in cardiovascular risk with the improvement of diabetic dyslipidemia. The ADA and AACE endorse the National Cholesterol Education Program Adult Treatment Program III (NCEP-ATP III) guidelines. (Table 4-5).[2,3,21] Because diabetes is considered a cardiovascular risk equivalent, the primary goal of therapy is a LDL cholesterol (LDL-C) level <100 mg/dL. In fact, the ADA recommends starting statin therapy to achieve a LDL-C reduction of 30% to 40% irrespective of baseline LDL-C levels in diabetics older than age 40. This recommendation is based primarily on the results of the Heart Protection Study (HPS), which showed a 25% reduction in the first event rate for major coronary events in individuals with diabetes older than age 40 and a total cholesterol level >135 mg/dL who received simvastatin (Zocor®) to achieve a LDL-C reduction of 30% from baseline.[22] For patients with diabetes and established CVD, or those considered at high risk for CVD, the LDL-C goal is <70 mg/dL.[23]

Because elevated Tgs and low HDL have been found to be independent markers for CVD, Tgs should be <150 mg/dL and HDL should be >40 mg/dL. For patients with Tgs ≥200 mg/dL despite reaching LDL-C goals, it is recommended to focus on a second lipid target known as non-HDL-cholesterol (non-HDL-C), which is equal to the total cholesterol level minus HDL cholesterol (HDL-C) and represents the atherogenic remnant lipoproteins, such as very-low-density lipoprotein (VLDL). The non-HDL-C goal is the LDL goal plus 30.[2]

## References

1.    Gaede P, Vedel P, Larsen N, et al: Multifactorial intervention and cardiovascular disease in patients with type 2 diabetes. *N Engl J Med* 2003;348:383-393.

2.    American Diabetes Association: Standards of medical care in diabetes—2007. *Diabetes Care* 2007;30(suppl 1):S4-S41.

3.    AACE Diabetes Mellitus Clinical Practice Guidelines Task Force: American Association of Clinical Endocrinologists medical guidelines for clinical practice for the management of diabetes mellitus. *Endocr Pract* 2007;13(suppl 1):S3-S68.

4.    The effect of intensive treatment of diabetes on the development and progression of long-term complications in insulin-dependent diabetes mellitus. The Diabetes Control and Complications Trial Research Group. *N Engl J Med* 1993;329:977-986.

5.    Nathan DM, Cleary PA, Backlund JY, et al, and the Diabetes Control and Complications Trial/Epidemiology of Diabetes Interventions and Complications (DCCT/EDIC) Study Research Group: Intensive diabetes treatment and cardiovascular disease in patients with type 1 diabetes. *N Engl J Med* 2005;353:2643-2653

6.   Intensive blood-glucose control with sulphonylureas or insulin compared with conventional treatment and risk of complications in patients with type 2 diabetes (UKPDS 33). UK Prospective Diabetes Study (UKPDS) Group. *Lancet* 1998;352:837-853.

7.   Ohkubo Y, Kishikawa H, Araki E, et al: Intensive insulin therapy prevents the progression of diabetic microvascular complications in Japanese patients with non-insulin-dependent diabetes mellitus: a randomized prospective 6-year study. *Diabetes Res Clin Pract* 1995;28:103-117.

8.   Garber AJ, Moghissi ES, Bransome ED, et al, and the American Endocrinology Task Force on Inpatient Diabetes and Metabolic Control: American College of Endocrinology position statement on inpatient diabetes and metabolic control. *Endocr Pract* 2004;10:77-82.

9.   Umpierrez GE, Isaacs SD, Bazargan N, et al: Hyperglycemia: an independent marker of in-hospital mortality in patients with undiagnosed diabetes. *J Clin Endocrinol Metab* 2002;87:978-982.

10.   Pomposelli JJ, Baxter JK, Babineau TJ, et al: Early postoperative glucose control predicts nosocomial infection rate in diabetic patients. *JPEN J Parenter Enteral Nutr* 1998;22:77-81.

11.   Kosiborod M, Rathore SS, Inzucchi SE, et al: Admission glucose and mortality in elderly patients hospitalized with acute myocardial infarction: implications for patients with and without recognized diabetes. *Circulation* 2005;111:3078-3086.

12.   Malmberg K, Norhammar A, Wedel H, et al: Glycometabolic state at admission: important risk marker of mortality in conventionally treated patients with diabetes mellitus and acute myocardial infarction; long-term results from the Diabetes and Insulin-Glucose Infusion in Acute Myocardial Infarction (DIGAMI) study. *Circulation* 1999;99:2626-2632.

13.   Furnary AP, Zerr KJ, Grunkemeier GL, et al: Continuous intravenous insulin infusion reduces the incidence of deep sternal wound infection in diabetic patients after cardiac surgical procedures. *Ann Thorac Surg* 1999;67:352-360; discussion 360-362.

14.   Furnary AP, Gao G, Grunkemeier GL, et al: Continuous insulin infusion reduces mortality in patients with diabetes undergoing coronary artery bypass grafting. *J Thorac Cardiovasc Surg* 2003;125:1007-1021.

15.   Lazar HL, Chipkin SR, Fitzgerald CA, et al: Tight glycemic control in diabetic coronary artery bypass graft patients improves

perioperative outcomes and decreases recurrent ischemic events. *Circulation* 2004;109:1497-1502.

16.   van den Berghe G, Wouters P, Weekers F, et al: Intensive insulin therapy in the critically ill patients. *N Engl J Med* 2001;345:1359-1367.

17.   van den Berghe G, Wilmer A, Hermans G, et al: Intensive insulin therapy in the medical ICU. *N Engl J Med* 2006;354:449-461.

18.   Krinsley J: Effect of intensive glucose management protocol on the mortality of critically ill adult patients. *Mayo Clin Proc* 2004;79:992-1000; erratum *Mayo Clin Proc* 2005;80:1101.

19.   ACOG technical bulletin. Diabetes and pregnancy. Number 200—December 1994 (replaces No. 92, May 1986). Committee on Technical Bulletins of the American College of Obstetricians and Gynecologists. *Int J Gynaecol Obstet* 1995;48:331-339.

20.   *National Diabetes Fact Sheet: United States 2005.* Available at: www.ndep.nih.gov/diabetes/pubs/2005_National_Diabetes_Fact_Sheet.pdf. Accessed July 21, 2007.

21.   *Third Report of the Expert Panel on the Detection, Evaluation, and Treatment of High Blood Cholesterol in Adults (Adult Treatment Panel III).* Available at: http://www.nhlbi.nih.gov/guidelines/cholesterol/index.htm. Accessed July 21, 2007.

22.   Collins R, Armitage J, Parish S, et al, and Heart Protection Study Collaborative Group: MRC/BHF Heart Protection Study of cholesterol-lowering with simvastatin in 5963 people with diabetes: a randomized placebo-controlled trial. *Lancet* 2003;361:2005-2016.

23.   Grundy SM, Cleeman JI, Merz CN, et al, and National Heart, Lung, and Blood Institute, American College of Cardiology Foundation, and American Heart Association: Implications of recent clinical trials for the National Cholesterol Education Program Adult Treatment Panel III guidelines. *Circulation* 2004;110:227-239.

# Chapter 5

# Lifestyle Considerations in Type 2 Diabetes Management

Medical nutrition therapy and exercise are integral components in both the prevention and management of type 2 diabetes. According to the American Diabetes Association (ADA), the goals of medical nutrition therapy are to decrease the risk of diabetes and cardiovascular disease (CVD) by promoting healthy food choices and physical activity, which should lead to moderate weight loss that is maintainable.[1] For patients with type 2 diabetes, the specific goals are to achieve and maintain glucose levels as close to normal as is safely possible, and a lipoprotein profile that reduces the risk for CVD and keeps blood pressure in the normal range. This should be accomplished while taking into account personal and cultural dietary preferences and only limiting food choices when supported by scientific evidence. Medical nutrition therapy is optimally provided by a registered dietitian who is educated in and familiar with the components of that therapy for the type 2 diabetes patient. For example, when dietitians provided basic or practice guideline based care to type 2 diabetes patients over a 6-month period, glycosylated hemoglobin $A_{1c}$ ($HbA_{1c}$) levels improved significantly compared with the control group, which did not work with a dietitian.[2] Common features of successful interventions include individualized programs, close contact with educators, education in self-management skills, use of behavioral change techniques, and frequent follow-up.[3] This chapter will briefly review some of the tenets of medical nutrition therapy and exercise in the management of type 2 diabetes.

## Macronutrients

No specific diets for diabetes have been endorsed by the ADA or American Association of Clinical Endocrinologists (AACE). Although multiple studies have attempted to identify the optimal macronutrient mix for the diabetic diet, none has been identified. The best mix varies, depending on individual patient circumstances. The Dietary Reference Intake (DRI) Report for healthy adults recommends 45% to 65% of daily energy intake from carbohydrates, 10% to 35% from proteins, and <10% to 35% from fats.[1,4] No matter what final macronutrient mix is recommended, the diabetic's total caloric intake must be appropriate to achieve and maintain weight management goals.

Carbohydrates are usually the primary determinant of postprandial-glucose response. This response is affected by not only the amount of carbohydrate ingested but also by the type of carbohydrate, macronutrient mix of the meal, method of preparation, and patient-specific variables, such as available insulin and the degree of insulin resistance. Fat and fiber intake in a mixed meal delay the absorption of carbohydrates and blunt glycemic response. Protein has a minimal effect on carbohydrate absorption and may increase insulin response without increasing plasma-glucose concentrations in patients with type 2 diabetes. As a result, carbohydrates containing mixed macronutrient compositions are not recommended to treat acute hypoglycemic episodes.

Because diabetes is considered a cardiovascular risk equivalent, decreasing the dietary determinants of atherogenic lipoproteins is integral to reducing the risk of CVD. Dietary saturated fat should be limited to <7% of daily energy intake with <200 mg/day of cholesterol. There is no safe level of transfatty acid intake, and transfats should be eliminated from a type 2 diabetes patient's diet.

Diets high in monounsaturated and polyunsaturated fatty acids (ie, Mediterranean diet) have beneficial effects on plasma-lipid concentrations and may reduce mortality. In fact, the ADA recommends that diabetics consume two or more servings of fish each week to provide required $\omega$-3 polyunsaturated fatty acids.[1]

For patients with normal renal function, there is no evidence that protein intake should be modified. However, for diabetic patients with chronic kidney disease (CKD), there is evidence that restricting protein intake to 0.8 g/kg of body weight/day may improve renal function and is recommended by the ADA. Because of the paucity of long-term clinical trials, low-carbohydrate diets (restricting total carbohydrates to <130 g/day) are not recommended for the prevention or management of diabetes.

Finally, it is recommended that diabetics adopt the US Department of Agriculture (USDA) recommended intake for dietary fiber (14 g of fiber/1,000 kcal). Clinical data suggest that dietary fiber reduces glycemia in type 1 diabetes patients and hyperinsulinemia, lipemia, and glycemia in type 2 diabetes patients.[4]

## Micronutrients

There is no definitive evidence to support vitamin supplementation in patients with type 2 diabetes unless they have specific vitamin deficiencies. Routine supplementation with antioxidants is not recommended because there is a lack of evidence supporting their benefit as well as concerns regarding their long-term safety. Benefits from chromium supplementation in diabetic management have not been consistently demonstrated and, therefore, chromium supplements are not recommended.

## Alcohol

The effect of alcohol on plasma-glucose levels depends on several variables including the amount of alcohol ingested, food intake, and the individual patient's medications. When ingested alone, moderate alcohol consumption has minimal effects on glucose and insulin concentrations. However, alcohol should be consumed with food to avoid hypoglycemia in individuals taking insulin or insulin secretagogues.

## Preventing Type 2 Diabetes

Multiple national and international trials, including the Diabetes Prevention Program (DPP), the Da Qing trial, and the Finnish Diabetes Prevention Study (FDPS), support diet and exercise as the most effective method for preventing type 2 diabetes.[5-7] Lifestyle modifications that include moderate weight loss (7% of body weight) and regular physical activity (150 min/week) can reduce the risk of developing type 2 diabetes and are recommended by the ADA, the AACE, and the American College of Endocrinology (ACE). No nutritional recommendations can be made for preventing type 1 diabetes.

## Recommended Lifestyle Modifications for Type 2 Diabetes Patients

Individuals with type 2 diabetes should be encouraged to make lifestyle modifications in an attempt to improve glycemia, dyslipidemia, and reduce their blood pressure and overall cardiovascular risk. These lifestyle changes should include reducing the intake of saturated and transfatty acids, cholesterol, and sodium, and increasing physical activity. A diet rich in fruits, vegetables, whole grains, nuts, and fiber may improve dyslipidemia, lower blood pressure, and decrease the risk of CVD.[8] Patients should learn how to limit carbohydrate consumption by either calculating the carbohydrate content of each meal based on grams of carbohydrate in commonly consumed foods or switching servings of foods based on carbohydrate unit equivalents from exchange lists. For patients using insulin secretagogues or fixed daily doses of insulin, carbohydrate intake should be consistent with respect to time of day and amount consumed on a daily basis.

## Recommended Lifestyle Modifications for Type 1 Diabetes Patients

Type 1 diabetes patients should be educated on estimating the carbohydrate content in their diets, so that they can accurately match mealtime insulin administration to carbohydrate intake by using insulin-to-carbohydrate ratios. Various methods are available for estimating carbohydrate intake, including experience-based estimation, the exchange system, and carbohydrate counting. No clinical trials have shown the superiority of one method over another. For patients using fixed daily doses of insulin, carbohydrate intake should be consistent with respect to time of day and amount consumed on a daily basis.

For planned exercise, patients should reduce their premeal bolus based on their level of anticipated activity to prevent hypoglycemia. Moderately intense exercise has been shown to increase glucose use by 2 to 3 mg/kg/min above usual requirements.[4] For example, a 70 kg person would need an additional 10 to 15 g of carbohydrates during moderate physical activity. More intense exercise would require the intake of more carbohydrates. As a result, unplanned physical activity usually requires supplemental carbohydrate intake to prevent hypoglycemia.

## Gestational Type 2 Diabetes

All women with gestational type 2 diabetes should receive medical nutrition therapy at the time of diagnosis. Medical nutrition therapy should focus on food choices that allow for adequate energy intake to provide appropriate weight gain, normoglycemia, and the absence of ketones. Weight loss during pregnancy is not recommended; however, obese or overweight women with gestational type 2 diabetes may benefit from modest exercise and carbohydrate restriction. Given the stringent glycemic targets suggested during pregnancy, the patient should monitor blood glucose frequently and maintain a dietary log that will provide valuable information for possible meal plan adjustments.

## Exercise

Regular exercise may prevent type 2 diabetes in high-risk individuals and has been shown to positively contribute to weight loss, improve glycemic control, improve cardiovascular risk factors, and improve a patient's physical well-being. The ADA recommends at least 150 min/week of moderate aerobic physical activity (50% to 70% of maximal heart rate) and resistance exercise that targets all major muscle groups 3 times/week. As with any treatment regimen, the effects of exercise must be thoroughly understood so that the benefits and risks can be analyzed for each patient and an exercise program appropriately designed.

### *Benefits of Exercise*

One exercise session often causes an acute decrease in plasma-glucose levels in type 2 diabetes patients. Postexercise enhancement of glucose metabolism, possibly from increased insulin sensitivity in muscle tissue, may last for hours or even days. However, more effective glycemic control may result from the additive effects of many exercise sessions and not from increased fitness.[9] Long-term studies have shown that regular exercise training consistently improves carbohydrate metabolism and insulin sensitivity and can maintain this effect for at least 5 years. In those studies, exercise intensity was 50% to 80% of maximum oxygen consumption, frequency was 3 to 4 times/week, and exercise duration was 30 to 60 min/session. $HbA_{1c}$ decreased 10% to 20%, and improvement in $HbA_{1c}$ levels was most pronounced in patients with mild disease as well as in the most insulin-resistant patients. This finding is consistent with the observation that physical exercise lessens insulin resistance.[10]

In patients with type 2 diabetes, most excess morbidity and mortality can be attributed to coronary artery disease (CAD), stroke, and peripheral vascular disease (PVD); all of these conditions are caused by accelerated atherosclerosis. Reducing atherogenesis is particularly crucial in these patients.[9] Hyperinsulinemia, hyperglycemia, and the insulin resistance syndrome are also increasingly seen as important risk factors for premature coronary disease in type 2 diabetes patients. The benefits of exercise in lowering cardiovascular risk are likely related to improved insulin sensitivity.[10] In patients with type 2 diabetes, decreases in adiposity frequently increase insulin sensitivity and glycemic control, and reduce risk factors for coronary heart disease (CHD). Weight loss and its maintenance are enhanced by combining exercise with dietary changes, and exercise disproportionately decreases intra-abdominal fat, which is the type of fat most closely associated with metabolic abnormalities. Exercise training is also associated with decreased anxiety, improved mood, higher self-esteem, and an increased sense of physical well-being, which may improve compliance with other therapies that enhance glycemic control.[9]

## Recommendations and Precautions

Pre-exercise evaluation of all diabetic patients is required. The clinician should obtain a complete patient history and perform an extensive physical examination, paying special attention to identifying macrovascular, microvascular, and neurologic complications that may put the patient at greater risk from exercise. Recommendations on the appropriate tests to pursue and precautions to follow for specific diabetic complications can be found in the ADA position statement on diabetes and exercise.[10]

If there are no contraindications to certain types of exercise, the type of exercise undertaken is a matter of patient preference. Rhythmic aerobic exercises, such as swimming and walking, are generally preferred. Resistance exercises, like weight lifting, may improve glucose disposal, but resistance exercise may also result in orthopedic and vascular problems. However, studies have shown that properly designed resistance exercise programs may be safer and more effective than assumed. High-resistance exercise using weights may be safe for young, healthy diabetic patients, but not for older patients or for those with long-standing disease. Moderate weight training programs using light weights and high numbers of repetitions can be used to maintain or enhance upper-body strength in almost all diabetic patients. Studies indicate that elderly patients benefit from exercise at least as much as the general population and that the incidence of complications in this group is at an acceptable level. An important caveat is that exercise may cause or worsen hypoglycemia in some patients, particularly those taking sulfonylureas (chlorpropamide [Diabinese®], glimepiride [Amaryl®], glipizide [Glucotrol®], glipizide extended-release [Glucotrol XL®], glyburide [DiaBeta®, Micronase®], micronized glyburide [Glynase® PresTab®], tolazamide [Tolinase®], tolbutamide) or insulin.[9] This may necessitate a reduction in the sulfonylurea or insulin dose or the addition of a carbohydrate snack before exercise.

## References

1.    Standards of medical care in diabetes—2007. *Diabetes Care* 2007;30(suppl 1):S4-S41. Available at: http://care.diabetesjournals.org/cgi/content/full/30/suppl_1/s4. Accessed August 14, 2007.

2.    Franz MJ, Monk A, Barry B, et al: Effectiveness of medical nutrition therapy provided by dietitians in the management of non-insulin-dependent diabetes mellitus: a randomized, controlled clinical trial. *J Am Diet Assoc* 1995;95:1009-1017.

3.    Agurs-Collins TD, Kumanyika SK, Ten Have TR, et al: A randomized controlled trial of weight reduction and exercise for diabetes management in older African-American subjects. *Diabetes Care* 1997;20:1503-1511.

4.    American Association of Clinical Endocrinologists medical guidelines for clinical practice for the management of diabetes mellitus. AACE Diabetes Mellitus Clinical Practice Guidelines Task Force. *Endocr Pract* 2007;13(suppl 1):S1-S68.

5.    Knowler WC, Barrett-Connor E, Fowler SE, et al, and the Diabetes Prevention Program Research Group: Reduction in the incidence of type 2 diabetes with lifestyle intervention or metformin. *N Engl J Med* 2002;346:393-403.

6.   Tuomilehto J, Lindstrom J, Eriksson J, et al, and the Finnish Diabetes Prevention Study Group: Prevention of type 2 diabetes mellitus by changes in lifestyle among subjects with impaired glucose tolerance. *N Engl J Med* 2001;344:1343-1350.

7.   Pan XR, Li GW, Hu YH, et al: Effects of diet and exercise in preventing NIDDM in people with impaired glucose tolerance. The Da Qing IGT and Diabetes Study. *Diabetes Care* 1997;20:537-544.

8.   Sacks FM, Svetkey LP, Vollmer WM, et al: Effects on blood pressure of reduced dietary sodium and the Dietary Approaches to Stop Hypertension (DASH) diet. DASH-Sodium Collaborative Research Group. *N Engl J Med* 2001;344:3-10.

9.   Exercise and NIDDM. *Diabetes Care* 1990;13:785-789.

10.   American Diabetes Association: Diabetes mellitus and exercise (Position Statement). *Diabetes Care* 2001;24(suppl 1):S51-S55.

5

# Chapter **6**

# Oral Hypoglycemic Agents

The therapeutic goal of diabetes management is to achieve a glycosylated hemoglobin $A_{1c}$ ($HbA_{1c}$) level as close to the normal range (4% to 6%) as possible, and at least <6.5%; this generally requires achieving a fasting plasma glucose (FPG) of <110 mg/dL, and a 2-hour postprandial plasma glucose (PPG) of <140 mg/dL.[1] These biochemical targets confer benefits in the reduction of diabetic complications, eg, nephropathy, neuropathy, and retinopathy. In addition, there is also a reduction in cardiovascular morbidity and mortality. Unfortunately, diabetes is still a chronic and progressive disease, which requires life-long pharmacotherapy in addition to diet and exercise.

Oral antidiabetics are prescribed for the treatment of type 2 diabetes to achieve and maintain near-normoglycemia as monotherapy or combination therapy, depending upon the patient's insulin reserve and level of insulin resistance at the time of diagnosis. This chapter briefly discusses the currently available oral antidiabetic agents and their indications, mechanisms of action, adverse effects, and contraindications.

At the present time, the following classes of oral antidiabetic agents are available in the United States:

- Biguanides
- Sulfonylureas
- Thiazolidinediones (TZDs)

- α-Glycosidase inhibitors
- Dipeptidyl peptidase IV (DPP-IV) inhibitors

## Biguanides

Metformin (Glucophage®, Glucophage® XR, Glumetza™) is the only available biguanide in the United States. It was first introduced in 1957 in France as an oral agent for therapy of type 2 diabetes, either used alone or in conjunction with sulfonylureas. Metformin received US Food and Drug Administration (FDA) approval in 1995.

### Mechanism of Action

Metformin's exact mechanism of action remains unclear. It reduces both FPG and the degree of postprandial hyperglycemia in patients with type 2 diabetes, but it has no effect on FPG in normal subjects.[2]

Metformin primarily increases insulin sensitivity in the liver by inhibiting hepatic gluconeogenesis, thereby reducing hepatic glucose production.[3] It also increases peripheral insulin sensitivity through mechanisms that are not fully understood.[4]

### Indications

Metformin is indicated as an adjunct to diet and exercise to improve glycemic control in patients with type 2 diabetes. Regular metformin is indicated in patients of at least 10 years of age; its extended-release form (Glucophage® XR) is indicated for use in patients of at least 17 years of age.[4] Because metformin is associated with weight loss, it is the first-line therapy for obese type 2 diabetes patients.[5] In diabetic patients, metformin provides cardiovascular protection that cannot be attributed to its antihyperglycemic effects. It should be initiated with a single dose, ie, usually 500 mg, taken with the biggest meal of the day to avoid any gastrointestinal (GI) side effects. Dosage increments can be made every 1 to 2 weeks up to a maximum daily dosage of 2,550 mg. The antidiabetic effect of metformin is dose dependent, and a plateau is reached at a daily dosage of 2,000 mg.

### Efficacy as a Monotherapy

Metformin is an insulin-sensitizing agent. In conjunction with diet, metformin reduces FPG concentration by 50 to 70 mg/dL, which corresponds to a 1.3% to 2% reduction in $HbA_{1c}$ levels. The magnitude of plasma-glucose reduction is related to pretreatment glucose levels. The efficacy of metformin monotherapy is independent of age, body weight, ethnicity, duration of the diabetes, insulin, or C-peptide level.[6]

### Efficacy as a Combination Therapy

Given the progressive nature of type 2 diabetes, combination therapy has evolved as standard practice especially after the United Kingdom Prospective Diabetes Study (UKPDS) trial findings indicated the superior control of glycemia with combination therapy vs monotherapy ($HbA_{1c}$ value, 7.5% vs 8.1%).[7] Metformin has been shown to be effective in combination with sulfonylureas, TZDs, insulin, and DPP-IV inhibitors. The maximum reduction of $HbA_{1c}$ achieved with any combination of oral antidiabetic drugs is 3% to 4%.

### Adverse Effects

GI side effects (ie, nausea, anorexia, abdominal bloating/cramping, diarrhea) are common in patients taking metformin and occur in 20% to 30% of patients. These side effects are usually mild and transient, and they can be minimized by slow dosage titration and dosage with food. About 5% of patients cannot tolerate metformin as the result of its GI side effects.[8] The probable etiology of these GI side effects may be a functional change in intestinal mucosa. Other clinically significant adverse effects include metallic taste and vitamin $B_{12}$ deficiency (10% to 30%), which are rarely of any clinical significance.

Metformin may increase plasma-lactate levels and precipitate the onset of lactic acidosis. The estimated incidence of metformin use resulting in lactic acidosis is 0.03 cases/1,000 patient-years.[5] Plasma concentration of metformin has no role in the development of lactic acidosis. Development of lactic acidosis is almost always related to the level of hypoxic conditions, ie, symptomatic congestive heart failure (CHF) or chronic obstructive pulmonary disease (COPD). Use of alcohol in large quantities may also potentiate the development of lactic acidosis in patients using metformin.

## Contraindications and Precautions

Metformin is contraindicated in patients with renal or hepatic disease, alcohol abuse syndrome, symptomatic CHF, respiratory insufficiency, dehydration, sepsis, or any acute illness that is associated with hypotension or hypoperfusion. Metformin is contraindicated if the patient's serum creatinine concentration is >1.4 mg/dL in women or 1.5 mg/dL in men or the glomerular filtration rate (GFR) is <70 mL/min in either sex.

Any patient undergoing radiocontrast studies should have metformin withheld 1 day before the study and 48 hours after the study to avoid any potential for lactic acidosis.

Use of metformin during pregnancy should be avoided. Metformin is classified as a Category B drug by the FDA. Category B drugs include prenatal vitamins, acetaminophen, and several other medications used routinely and safely during pregnancy. If there is a clinical need for a Category B drug, it is considered safe to use it. In pregnant diabetic women, insulin is still recommended as the best treatment. Metformin is excreted in the breast milk in miniscule concentration, and no clinical adverse events have been reported in infants of mothers taking metformin while breast feeding.[8]

## Sulfonylureas

Sulfonylureas are the most widely prescribed drugs for the treatment of type 2 diabetes.[9] Biochemical modification of the sulfonic acid-urea nucleus has resulted in the production of agents that have similar qualitative action, but different potencies (Table 6-1).[10] Sulfonylureas are divided into first- and second-generation groups based on the potency of the drug and its duration of action. All insulin secretagogues, except for their duration of actions, generally act the same; however, certain secretagogues have differences that may be clinically important. Chlorpropamide (Diabinese®) can cause serious hypoglycemia in patients with renal insufficiency and can also cause water intoxication syndrome; chlorpropamide is no longer widely prescribed.[11] Different preparations of glipizide (Glucotrol®, Glucotrol XL®) also have markedly different pharmacokinetics with different potencies. Five milligrams of extended-release glipizide (Glucotrol XL®) once daily is enough to provide full efficacy, compared with 10 mg, twice daily for conventional glipizide (Glucotrol®).[10] The most controversial issue regarding individual secretagogues concerns glyburide (DiaBeta®, Micronase®). In the University Group Diabetes Program (UGDP) study, glyburide use was associated with a decrease in myocardial ischemic preconditioning and has been given a black box warning by the FDA.[12,13]

### Indications

Sulfonylureas can be prescribed as monotherapy in the drug-naive type 2 diabetics and in combination with metformin, TZDs, and insulin.

### Mechanism of Action

The proposed mechanisms of action of sulfonylureas include the augmentation of insulin release from pancreatic β-cells and the potentiation of insulin's action on its target cells.

Sulfonylureas bind to a specific receptor on pancreatic β-cells. This binding is maximum for glyburide and minimum for tolbutamide. This binding also leads to activation of receptors with the resultant depolarization of β-cells. This depolarized state permits calcium to enter the cell and actively promote insulin release. These receptors consist of two proteins—a protein that binds the sulfonylurea-sulfonylurea receptor and an ATP-sensitive potassium channel.[9]

The extrapancreatic effects of sulfonylureas, eg, potentiation of the peripheral effects of insulin at the receptor or postreceptor level, have been acknowledged for their continued efficacy despite a lack of demonstrable increase in insulin secretion.[14] However, these effects are only limited to in vitro studies because clinical trials have failed to show any therapeutic benefit of sulfonylureas when added to insulin therapy in the patient with type 1 diabetes.[15]

## Efficacy as a Monotherapy

All sulfonylureas are equally effective in reducing plasma glucose. The choice of a sulfonylurea is primarily dependent upon its cost and availability; however, owing to the fear of inducing hypoglycemia, sulfonylureas with a short duration of action are preferred by most physicians. The potency of a sulfonylurea is directly related to a patient's initial FPG level; the higher the FPG level at baseline, the greater it will drop with treatment.

Predictors of a good response to sulfonylurea therapy include recently diagnosed type 2 diabetes, mild-to-moderate fasting hyperglycemia, a good β-cell function as indicated by a high C-peptide level, and the absence of islet cell or glutamic acid decarboxylase 65 (GAD65) antibodies. Most clinical trials have shown a maximum reduction of 20% in plasma-glucose concentrations or a drop in $HbA_{1c}$ of 1.5% to 2% with the use of a sulfonylurea as monotherapy compared with placebo.[16]

## Table 6-1: Secretagogues—Sulfonylureas and Nonsulfonylureas

| Generic Name | Approved Daily Dosage Range (mg) |
|---|---|
| **Sulfonylurea— *first generation*** | |
| Chlorpropamide (Diabinese®) | 100-500 (750 max) |
| Tolazamide (Tolinase®) | 100-1,000 |
| Tolbutamide | 500-3,000 |
| **Sulfonylurea— *second generation*** | |
| Glimepiride (Amaryl®) | 1-8 |
| Glipizide (Glucotrol®) | 2.5-40 |
| Glipizide (extended release) (Glucotrol XL®) | 5-10 (20 max) |
| Glyburide (DiaBeta®, Glynase®, Micronase®) | 1.25-20 |
| Glyburide (micronized) (Glynase® PresTab®) | 0.75-12 |
| **Nonsulfonylureas** | |
| Repaglinide (Prandin®) | 0.5-16 |
| Nateglinide (Starlix®) | 180-360 |

| Duration of Action (hr) | Clearance |
| --- | --- |
| >48 | Renal |
| 12-24 | Hepatic, renal |
| 6-12 | Hepatic |
| 24 | Hepatic, renal |
| 12-18 | Hepatic |
| 24 | Hepatic |
| 12-24 | Hepatic, renal |
| 12-24 | Hepatic, renal |
| 2-6 | Hepatic |
| 2-4 | Renal |

6

Diabetic patients who are not responsive to first-generation sulfonylureas (ie, chlorpropamide, tolbutamide) are less likely to be responsive to second-generation sulfonylureas (ie, glipizide, glipizide extended-release, glyburide, micronized glyburide [Glynase® PresTab®]). As a general rule, the glucose-lowering effect of sulfonylureas plateaus once half the maximum recommended dose is reached. After an initial adequate response to sulfonylureas, about 5% to 10% of patients will show a decline in their glycemic control (ie, secondary failure) and will require a second oral agent. Factors contributing to secondary failure include a progressive decline in β-cells, weight gain, lack of exercise, poor compliance, β-cell apoptosis, secondary conditions that affect the release of insulin, or an increase in insulin resistance.[17]

### Efficacy as a Combination Therapy

Sulfonylureas are available in combination with metformin and TZDs.

### Adverse Effects

Less than 2% of patients treated with sulfonylureas discontinue their treatment because of adverse side effects. The most common adverse side effect is hypoglycemia, which is more common with agents that have a longer duration of action, ie, chlorpropamide and glyburide. Severe hypoglycemia requiring hospitalization has been reported in the frequency of 0.2 to 0.4 cases/1,000 patient-years for sulfonylurea therapy, although the UKPDS reported an incidence of 1.2% in the sulfonylurea-treated group.[7] Hypoglycemia is most likely to occur during the initiation of sulfonyurea therapy. Other factors that predispose a patient to hypoglycemia include too high of a dose; missed meals; alcohol abuse; concomitant use of salicylates, sulfonamides, or fibric acid derivatives; and a history of renal, hepatic, or cardiovascular disease (CVD).[17]

Weight gain is another problematic adverse effect of sulfonylureas, especially if glycemic control improves substantially. However, in one study, glipizide extended-release caused no weight gain. Average weight gain on a sulfonylurea is 2 to 5 kg.[18]

Other infrequent adverse effects include GI disturbance, photosensitivity, abnormalities of liver enzymes, and flushing, especially when chlorpropamide is combined with alcohol. Chlorpropamide can also induce hyponatremia, particularly in patients on diuretics.[14] Sulfonylureas have been shown to have adverse effects on the cardiovascular system, especially in patients with pre-existing coronary artery disease (CAD). Studies have shown that sulfonylureas prevent ischemic preconditioning of the myocardium as a result of their ability to block potassium channels.[12]

### *Contraindications and Precautions*

Sulfonylureas are contraindicated in patients who are hypersensitive to glipizide or any component of the formulation, other sulfonamides, lactating, and who have insulin-dependent type 1 diabetes or diabetic ketoacidosis.

## Nonsulfonylurea Secretagogues

The nonsulfonylurea secretagogues repaglinide (Prandin®), a benzoic acid derivative, and nateglinide (Starlix®), a phenylalanine derivative, are similar in action to sulfonylureas because they act on the same β-cell receptors (Table 6-2). However, nonsulfonylurea secretagogues are distinguished from sulfonylureas by their short half-lives, and also because they do not contain sulfonic acid moiety and, therefore, are useful in patients who are allergic to sulfa drugs.[19] Nonsulfonylurea secretagogues are rapidly absorbed and eliminated, and cause a fast, but brief, release of insulin, resulting in attenuation of PPG excursions. Nateglinide has little stimulatory effect on insulin secretion when administered in the fasting state, thus minimizing the risk of hypoglycemia.[20]

## Table 6-2: Properties of Antihyperglycemic Agent Classes

|  | Secretagogues | Metformin |
|---|---|---|
| **Mechanism of action** | Potentiate insulin secretion | Suppresses liver glucose production |
| **HbA$_{1c}$ reduction (%) as monotherapy** | 1.5-2 | 1.5-2 |
| **Adverse effects** | Hypoglycemia, weight gain | Nausea, diarrhea, risk of lactic acidosis in renal insufficiency |
| **Nonglycemic effects** | None | Reduces cardiovascular risk markers; limits weight gain |
| **Evidence for benefit** | | |
| *Microvascular* | Strong | Strong |
| *Macrovascular* | None | Moderate |

AGIs=α-Glucosidase inhibitors; DFP-IV=dipeptidyl peptidase IVs; HbA$_{1c}$=glycosylated hemoglobin A$_{1c}$; TZDs=thiazolidinediones

| AGIs | TZDs | DPP-IVs |
|------|------|---------|
| Delay intestinal carbohydrate absorption | Improve insulin sensitivity (ie, fat, liver, muscle) | Potentiate glucose-dependent insulin release, suppress glucagon secretion |
| 0.5-1 | 0.75-2 | 0.79-0.94 |
| Flatulence, diarrhea | Edema, congestive heart failure (CHF), weight gain, anemia, fracture | Rare allergic reactions |
| Reduce cardiovascular risk markers | Reduce cardiovascular risk markers | Weight neutral, no hypoglycemia |
| None | None | None |
| Weak | Weak | None |

## Efficacy

The efficacy of repaglinide is similar to that of the sulfonylureas, but nateglinide appears to be less potent. Multiple comparative studies of repaglinide vs the sulfonylureas have shown equal efficacy; however, one study did find that metformin was superior to repaglinide in lowering glucose levels.

## Adverse Effects

Hypoglycemia and weight gain are the primary side effects of repaglinide and nateglinide therapy. These side effects are usually less pronounced than the side effects associated with sulfonylureas. Administering repaglinide and nateglinide only before meals further minimizes the risk of hypoglycemia. No clinically significant changes in liver enzymes or cardiovascular toxicity have been reported with repaglinide or nateglinide use.[21]

## Drug Interactions

The metabolism of repaglinide and nateglinide is inhibited by ketoconazole (Nizoral®) and erythromycin, and may actually be enhanced by drugs that induce the CYP3A4 isoenzyme. Both repaglinide and nateglinide are highly bound to plasma proteins (98%). Nonsteroidal anti-inflammatory drugs (NSAIDs), salicylates, monoamine oxidase (MAO) inhibitors, and nonselective β-blockers may potentiate the hypoglycemic effects of repaglinide and nateglinide, whereas thiazides, corticosteroids, and thyroid products may reduce those effects.[22]

## Contraindications and Precautions

Repaglinide and nateglinide are contraindicated in type 1 diabetes and in pregnancy. Both drugs are metabolized in the liver and should be used with caution in patients with liver disease. However, repaglinide and nateglinide are safe to use in patients with renal failure. Their hypoglycemic effect is potentiated with strenuous physical exercise, alcohol ingestion, insufficient caloric intake, and in combination with other oral hypoglycemic agents.[21]

## Thiazolidinediones

The introduction of TZDs has revolutionized type 2 diabetes management, despite the fact that the first TZD, troglitazone, was removed from the US market due to idiosyncratic hepatocellular injury. The TZDs pioglitazone (Actos®) and rosiglitazone (Avandia®) are currently available in the United States.

### *Mechanism of Action*

TZDs are selective agonists for the nuclear receptor peroxisome-proliferator-activated receptor-γ (PPAR-γ) (Table 6-2). The role of PPARs in humans is associated with the regulation of gene transcription by two mechanisms. The first mechanism is transactivation, a DNA-dependent pathway. After activation in the cytoplasm, PPARs bind to a retinoid X receptor/retinoic acid receptor. The formation of this complex allows PPARs to be transported into the nucleus of an atom and bind to the promoter region of the regulated gene. The second mechanism, transrepression, a DNA-independent pathway, interferes with other transcription pathways and may be responsible for the anti-inflammatory actions of TZDs.[23]

The intricate interactions of TZDs result in increased insulin-stimulated glucose uptake by skeletal muscle cells, decreased hepatic glucose production, decreased lipolysis, and enhanced adipocyte differentiation.[24]

### *Indications*

TZDs can be prescribed as monotherapy or in combination with metformin or sulfonylureas. The use of TZDs is not recommended in combination with insulin due to patient fears of excessive weight gain and fluid retention.

## Efficacy

In placebo-controlled trials, TZDs lower $HbA_{1c}$ as effectively as sulfonylureas and metformin. Many head-to-head studies comparing TZDs with metformin and sulfonylureas have shown equal reductions in $HbA_{1c}$.[25,26] Among the TZDs on the US market, rosiglitazone is more potent than pioglitazone. Its binding affinity for PPAR-$\gamma$ is approximately 30 times greater than that of pioglitazone, which means a clinical dose of rosiglitazone is about one sixth that of pioglitazone (4 to 8 mg vs 15 to 45 mg). In comparative studies, both rosiglitazone and pioglitazone have shown equal efficacy in lowering $HbA_{1c}$ level, although pioglitazone was more effective on triglycerides (Tgs) and other inflammatory markers.[27]

As monotherapy, clinical trials of TZDs have shown $HbA_{1c}$ reduction in the range of 0.3% to 1.6% in drug-naive patients. As combination therapy with sulfonylureas and metformin, the reduction in $HbA_{1c}$ is additive and sustained.[21]

The A Diabetes Outcome Progression Trial (ADOPT) was a large, international, multicenter trial designed to evaluate the long-term efficacy of monotherapy with rosiglitazone on glycemic control and progression of diabetes-associated pathophysiologic abnormalities in 4,300 recently diagnosed, treatment-naive type 2 diabetes patients.[28] Results of the study, which compared the efficacy of rosiglitazone monotherapy with metformin or glyburide monotherapy, demonstrated that initial treatment with rosiglitazone reduced the risk of monotherapy failure in these patients at 5 years by 32% compared with metformin and by 63% compared with glyburide. In addition, rosiglitazone was more effective than metformin or glyburide in delaying progressive loss of glycemic control, as measured by $HbA_{1c}$ and FPG levels. Rosiglitazone was shown to significantly improve insulin sensitivity and reduce the rate of loss of $\beta$-cell function vs the other two agents.

## Adverse Effects

The most commonly reported adverse effects of TZDs are upper respiratory tract infections (16%) and headache (7.1%).[29] These effects are mild and transient in the majority of patients and usually do not necessitate the discontinuation of the medication.

The most unpleasant adverse effect for the patient is weight gain, which ranges from 3 to 5 kg. The weight gain associated with TZDs appears to involve peripheral subcutaneous sites with a reduction in visceral fat depot.[30] Edema can also occur because of the activation of PPAR receptors in the kidneys, which leads to fluid retention. This fluid retention can precipitate CHF in patients with compromised cardiac function.[31] Anemia may occur infrequently and is considered to be dilutional in nature.[32]

Recent safety analyses of the ADOPT cohort and the Prospective Pioglitazone Clinical Trial in Macrovascular Events (PROactive) cohort showed an increased incidence of distal extremity fractures only in postmenopausal women who were prescribed rosiglitazone and pioglitazone, respectively.[33] Other risk factors for fracture with TZDs are currently under investigation.

TZDs are extremely safe in terms of liver toxicity; only 12 reports of hepatotoxicity with rosiglitazone and pioglitazone have been reported.[17]

## Contraindications and Precautions

TZDs should be used with caution in patients with established liver disease. Liver transaminases should be checked before initiation of treatment, and treatment with TZDs should not be initiated in patients with transaminases that are more than 2.5 times the upper limit. A patient's alanine aminotransferase (ALT) level should be monitored every 2 months for the first year and periodically thereafter. If the ALT level increases more than three times the upper limit of normal, TZD therapy should be discontinued.[17]

TZDs should be used with caution in patients with symptomatic CHF (New York Heart Association [NYHA] classifications 1 and 2) and are contraindicated in NYHA classes 3 and 4. TZDs should also be used with caution in patients with peripheral edema because their use may worsen the edema.[31]

Premenopausal, infertile women may experience resumption of ovulation while on TZDs, and they should be cautioned about the possibility of unexpected pregnancy. TZDs are contraindicated during pregnancy and lactation.[17]

## α-Glucosidase Inhibitors

α-Glucosidase inhibitors do not target any specific pathophysiologic defect of type 2 diabetes (Table 6-2). Instead, α-glucosidase inhibitors delay the absorption of complex carbohydrates, and thus inhibit PPG peaks and consequently lower postprandial-insulin levels. Currently, two α-glucosidase inhibitors are available in the United States—acarbose (Precose®) and miglitol (Glyset®). Emiglitate and voglibose, two other α-glucosidase inhibitors, are not currently available in the United States. In the treatment of type 2 diabetes, α-glucosidase inhibitors have been proven to have beneficial effects on glycemic control and postload-insulin levels, but there is no evidence of a reduction in mortality or morbidity with the use of α-glucosidase inhibitors.[34]

### *Mechanism of Action*

An enzyme in the brush border of the proximal small intestinal epithelium, α-glucosidase breaks down disaccharides and other complex carbohydrates to simple absorbable glucose. α-Glucosidase inhibitors are competitive inhibitors of this enzyme and delay the absorption of glucose, thus inhibiting PPG excursions and lowering postprandial-insulin levels. The overall absorption of carbohydrates is not reduced by the use of α-glucosidase.[21]

## Efficacy

α-Glucosidase inhibitors are less effective than any other class of oral hypoglycemic agents in reducing FPG, resulting in a decrease of 20 to 30 mg/dL. These inhibitors also reduce the $HbA_{1c}$ levels by 0.5% to 1%. The primary effect of α-glucosidase inhibitors is on PPG levels, resulting in a decrease of 40 to 60 mg/dL.[17] Type 2 diabetics who consume >50% of their daily calories as carbohydrates show the greatest reduction in $HbA_{1c}$. In the UKPDS, approximately 2,000 patients on dietary, sulfonylurea, metformin, or insulin therapy were randomized to acarbose or placebo. At the end of 3 years, 60% of the patients in the UKPDS had discontinued taking acarbose mostly because of adverse GI side effects. The 40% of patients who remained on acarbose showed a $HbA_{1c}$ reduction of 0.5% compared with placebo. In another meta-analysis, acarbose dosages >50 mg three times daily did not confer any additional glycemic benefit, but were associated with more adverse side effects.[35]

## Adverse Effects

GI side effects are the primary reason for patients to discontinue the use of acarbose or miglitol. These side effects include flatulence, abdominal discomfort, and diarrhea. Taking a tablet with the first bite of each meal can minimize these adverse effects. High doses of acarbose (ie, 200 to 300 mg three times daily) may result in elevated serum aminotransferase levels that resolve with discontinuation of the drug.

Hypoglycemia also may result when α-glucosidase inhibitors are used in combination with sulfonylureas or insulin. Ingesting glucose itself, as opposed to more complex carbohydrates, reverses hypoglycemia in this setting.[29]

## Drug Interactions

Miglitol decreases the bioavailability of ranitidine (Zantac®) and propranolol (Inderal®, Inderal® LA) by 50% in healthy volunteers.[36]

### Contraindications and Precautions

Use of acarbose is contraindicated in cirrhosis of the liver, whereas miglitol is contraindicated in renal failure.[37] α-Glucosidase inhibitors are also contraindicated in patients with inflammatory bowel disease (IBD) because they precipitate pre-existing diarrhea. Both acarbose and miglitol are rated Category B during pregnancy.[38]

## Dipeptidyl Peptidase IV Inhibitors

Glucagon-like peptide-1 (GLP-1) is an insulinotropic hormone secreted by L-cells of the small intestine. GLP-1 has several important biologic actions including the stimulation of insulin secretion in a glucose-dependent manner, inhibition of gastric emptying, suppression of glucagon secretion, and central anorexic activity.

Patients with type 2 diabetes exhibit reduced levels of active GLP-1 (amino acids 7 to 36) along with an impaired GLP-1 response to a glucose load. Endogenous GLP-1 also has undesirable pharmacokinetics; after it is secreted, it is rapidly cleaved and inactivated (ie, plasma half-life <1 min) by the enzyme DPP-IV. This understanding of diabetes pathophysiology led to the introduction of a new class of therapeutics for diabetes management known as DPP-IV inhibitors. The DPP-IV inhibitors, unlike other GLP-1-based therapies (ie, exenatide [Byetta®]), can be administered orally.[39]

A number of DPP-IV inhibitors are under evaluation by the pharmaceutical industry, but only sitagliptin (Januvia™) has been approved by the FDA for the treatment of type 2 diabetes, as monotherapy or in combination therapy with metformin or a TZD.

### Efficacy

DPP-IV inhibitors lower $HbA_{1c}$ 0.79% to 0.94% as monotherapy.[39,40] In an individual trial, sitagliptin was found to be as efficacious as glipizide.[41] Sitagliptin lowers both FPG and PPG.

### Nonglycemic Outcomes

DPP-IV inhibitors are considered weight neutral when compared with sulfonylureas and TZDs.[42]

Some studies have shown a slight improvement in patient lipid profiles with DPP-IV inhibitors compared with TZDs and metformin.[40-42]

### Adverse Effects

Overall, DPP-IV inhibitors are well tolerated with few adverse side effects. The most common adverse effects include nasopharyngitis, increased risk of UTI, and headache.[42] Infrequently, allergic reactions have been attributed to sitagliptin, including rare cases of angioedema and Stevens-Johnson syndrome (SJS). Consistent with their mechanism of action, use of DPP-IV inhibitors is not associated with hypoglycemia unless combined with a sulfonylurea or insulin.

### Precautions

The usual dose of sitagliptin is 100 mg once daily, which is reduced to 50 mg for moderate-to-severe renal insufficiency (GFR <30 to 50 mL/min) and 25 mg for severe renal insufficiency (<30 mL/min).[40]

## References

1.  ACE Consensus Conference on Guidelines for Glycemic Control. Available at: http://www.aace.com/meetings/consensus/dcc/pdf/supplementv8s1.pdf. Accessed August 8, 2007.

2.  Inzucchi ES: Oral antihyperglycemic therapy for type 2 diabetes: scientific review. *JAMA* 2002;287:360-372.

3.  Bailey CJ, Turner RC: Metformin. *N Eng J Med* 1996;334:574-579.

4.  Johansen K: Efficacy of metformin in the treatment of NIDDM. Meta-analysis. *Diabetes Care* 1999;22:33-37.

5.  Hundal RS, Krssak M, Dufour S, et al: Mechanism by which metformin reduces glucose production in type 2 diabetes. *Diabetes* 2000;49:2063-2069.

6. Cusi K, DeFronzo RA: Metformin: a review of its metabolic effects. *Diabetes Rev* 1999;6:89-130.

7. UK Prospective Diabetes Study (UKPDS) Group: Effect of intensive blood-glucose control with metformin on complications in overweight patients with type 2 diabetes (UKPDS 34). *Lancet* 1998;352:854-865; erratum *Lancet* 1998;352:854-865.

8. Misbin RI, Green L, Stadel BV, et al: Lactic acidosis in patients with diabetes treated with metformin. *N Eng J Med* 1998;338: 265-266.

9. Zimmerman BR: Sulfonylureas. *Endocrin Metab Clin North Am* 1997;26:511-522.

10. Simonson DC, Kourides IA, Feinglos M, et al: Efficacy, safety, and dose-response characteristics of glipizide gastrointestinal therapeutic system on glycemic control and insulin secretion in NIDDM. Results of two multicenter, randomized, placebo-controlled clinical trials. The Glipizide Gastrointestinal Therapeutic System Study Group. *Diabetes Care* 1997;20:597-606.

11. Chaudhry ZW, Gannon MC, Nuttall FQ: Stability of body weight in type 2 diabetes *Diabetes Care* 2006;29:493-497.

12. Meinert CL, Knatterud GL, Prout TE, et al: A study of the effects of hypoglycemic agents on vascular complications in patients with adult-onset diabetes. II. Mortality results. *Diabetes* 1970;19(suppl):789-830.

13. Lee TM, Chou TF: Impairment of myocardial protection in type 2 diabetic patients. *J Clin Endocrinol Metab* 2003;88:531-537.

14. Aguilar-Bryan L, Nichols CG, Wechsler SW, et al: Cloning of the beta cell high-affinity sulfonylurea receptor: a regulator of insulin secretion. *Science* 1995;268:423-426.

15. Kaku K, Inoue Y, Kaneko T: Extrapancreatic effects of sulfonylurea drugs. *Diabetes Res Clin Pract* 1995;28(suppl):S105-S108.

16. Cheng AY, Fantus IG: Oral antihyperglycemic therapy for type 2 diabetes mellitus. *CMAJ* 2005;172:213-226.

17. Davis SN: Insulin, hypoglycemic agents, and the pharmacology of the endocrine pancreas. In: Brunton LL, Lazo JS, Parker KL, et al, eds: *Goodman & Gilman's The Pharmacological Basis of Therapeutics*, 11th ed. McGraw Hill, New York, NY, 2006, pp 1613-1646.

18. Stenman S, Melander A, Groop PH, et al: What is the benefit of increasing the sulfonylurea dose? *Ann Intern Med* 1993;118: 169-172.

19. Blickle JF: Meglitinide analogues: a review of clinical data focused on recent trials. *Diabetes Metab* 2006;32:113-120.

20. Rosenstock J, Hassman DR, Madder RD, et al, and the Repaglinide Versus Nateglinide Comparison Study Group: Repaglinide versus nateglinide monotherapy: a randomized, multicenter study. *Diabetes Care* 2004;27:1265-1270.

21. Levetan C: Oral antidiabetic agents in type 2 diabetes. *Curr Med Res Opin* 2007;23:945-952.

22. Scheen AJ: Drug interactions of clinical importance with antihyperglycaemic agents: an update. *Drug Saf* 2005;28:601-631.

23. Yki-Jarvinen H: Thiazolidinediones. *N Engl J Med* 2004;351: 1106-1118.

24. Iwamoto Y, Kosaka K, Kuzuya T, et al: Effects of troglitazone: a new hypoglycemic agent in patients with NIDDM poorly controlled by diet therapy. *Diabetes Care* 1996;19:151-156.

25. Kahn SE, Haffner SM, Heise MA, et al, and the ADOPT Study Group: Glycemic durability of rosiglitazone, metformin, or glyburide monotherapy. *N Engl J Med* 2006;355:2427-2443.

26. Waugh J, Keating GM, Plosker GL, et al: Pioglitazone: a review of its use in type 2 diabetes mellitus. *Drugs* 2006;66:85-109.

27. Berhanu P, Kipnes MS, Khan MA, et al: Effect of pioglitazone on lipid and lipoprotein profiles in patients with type 2 diabetes and dyslipidaemia after treatment conversion from rosiglitazone while continuing stable statin therapy. *Diab Vasc Dis Res* 2006;3:39-44.

28. Kahn SE, Haffner SM, Heise MA, et al: Glycemic durability of rosiglitazone, metformin, or glyburide monotherapy. *N Engl J Med* 2006;355:2427-2443.

29. Spiller HA, Sawyer TS: Toxicology of oral antidiabetic medications. *Am J Health Syst Pharm* 2006;63:929-938.

30. Jacob AN, Salinas K, Adams-Huet B, et al: Weight gain in type 2 diabetes mellitus. *Diabetes Obes Metab* 2007;9:386-393.

31. Granberry MC, Hawkins JB, Franks AM: Thiazolidinediones in patients with type 2 diabetes mellitus and heart failure. *Am J Health Syst Pharm* 2007;64:931-936.

**6**

32.   Lindenfeld J, Masoudi FA: Fluid retention with thiazolidine-diones: does the mechanism influence the outcome? *J Am Coll Cardiol* 2007;49:1705-1707.

33.   Ruder K: Type 2 drug up risk of fractures. *Diabetes Forecast* 2007;60:29-30.

34.   Van de Laar FA, Lucassen PL, Rutten GE, et al: Alpha-gluco-sidase inhibitors for type 2 diabetes mellitus. *Cochrane Database Syst Rev* 2005;(2):CD003639.

35.   Van de Laar FA, Lucassen PL, Akkermans RP, et al: Alpha-glucosidase inhibitors for patients with type 2 diabetes: results from a Cochrane systemic review and meta-analysis. *Diabetes Care* 2005;28:154-163.

36.   Glyset® Package Insert. Pfizer Inc. New York, NY, 2006.

37.   Andrade RJ, Lucena MI, Rodriguez-Mendizabal M: Hepatic injury caused by acarbose. *Ann Intern Med* 1996;124:931.

38.   Catalan VS, Couture JA, LeLorier J: Predictors of persistence of use of the novel antidiabetic agent acarbose. *Arch Intern Med* 2001;161:1106-1112.

39.   Aschner P, Williams-Herman DE, Lunceford JK, et al, and the Sitagliptin Study 021 Group: Effect of the dipeptidyl peptidase-4 inhibitor sitagliptin as monotherapy on glycemic control in patients with type 2 diabetes. *Diabetes Care* 2006;29:2632-2637.

40.   Scott R, Wu M, Sanchez M, et al: Efficacy and tolerability of the dipeptidyl peptidase-4 inhibitor sitagliptin as monotherapy over 12 weeks in patients with type 2 diabetes. *Int J Clin Pract* 2007;61:171-180.

41.   Nauck MA, Meininger G, Sheng D, et al, and the Sitagliptin Study 024 Group: Efficacy and safety of the dipeptidyl peptidase-4 inhibitor, sitagliptin, compared with the sulfonylurea, glipizide, in patients with type 2 diabetes inadequately controlled on metformin alone: a randomized, double blind, non-inferiority trial. *Diabetes Obes Metab* 2007;9:194-205.

42.   Amori ER, Lau J, Pittas AG: Efficacy and safety of incretin therapy in type 2 diabetes: systematic review and meta-analysis. *JAMA* 2007;298:194-206.

# Chapter 7

# Parenteral Therapies in Type 2 Diabetes

## Insulin Therapy

Insulin is the most studied and ultimately the most effective agent for treating type 2 diabetes. Many patients will require insulin therapy at some point because oral hypoglycemic agents eventually fail to adequately control progressive hyperglycemia. The United Kingdom Prospective Diabetes Study (UKPDS) showed that about 30% of newly diagnosed patients taking sulfonylureas (glimepiride [Amaryl®], glyburide [DiaBeta®, Micronase®], micronized glyburide [Glynase® PresTab®], glipizide [Glucotrol®, Glucotrol XL®]) and 22% of those taking metformin (Glucophage®, Glucophage® XR, Glumetza™) required insulin within 6 years because oral agents failed to maintain control.[1]

Insulins are divided for practical purposes into two broad categories, basal and bolus, based on their pharmacokinetics.

### Basal Insulin

Basal insulin refers to exogenous insulin per unit of time that is necessary to prevent unchecked gluconeogenesis and ketogenesis. It provides a constant background level of insulin that controls plasma glucose overnight while the patient sleeps and between meals when they are not eating and the meal bolus insulin action has waned. When dosed

## Table 7-1: Basal and Bolus Insulin Pharmacokinetics

| Category of Insulin | Generic Name | Brand Name |
| --- | --- | --- |
| Long-acting (preferred) | Glargine | Lantus® |
| | Detemir | Levemir® |
| Intermediate-acting | NPH | Humulin® N, Novolin® N |
| Rapid-acting | Lispro | Humalog® |
| | Aspart | NovoLog® |
| | Glulisine | Apidra® |
| Short-acting (regular) | Regular insulin | Humulin® R, Novolin® R |
| Inhaled insulin | Inhaled insulin | Exubera® |

NPH=Neutral Protamine Hagedorn

appropriately, basal insulin should not cause hypoglycemia if the patient does not eat or ingests less food than anticipated during a meal. Available basal insulins include glargine (Lantus®), detemir (Levemir®), and Neutral Protamine Hagedorn (NPH). Basal insulin can also be provided by rapid-acting insulin or short-acting (regular) (Humulin® R, Novolin® R) insulin delivered subcutaneously via an insulin pump.

Basal insulins for subcutaneous injection may be broadly categorized into long-acting (ie, glargine, detemir) and intermediate-acting (ie, NPH) insulins. The salient features of each currently available basal insulin are described below and summarized in (Table 7-1).

| Time to Onset | Time to Peak | Duration of Action (hr) |
|---|---|---|
| 2-4 hr | No pronounced peak | 20-24 |
| 2 hr | No pronounced peak | 6-24 |
| 2-4 hr | 4-10 hr | 12-18 |
| 5-15 min | 30-90 min | 4-6 |
| 30-60 min | 2-4 hr | 6-8 |
| 7 min | 1 hr | 4-8 |

*Insulin glargine:* Glargine is a recombinant human insulin analogue. It differs from human insulin in that asparagine at position A21 is replaced by glycine, and two arginines are added to the C terminus of the β chain. Because of these changes, insulin glargine is soluble in an acidic environment and forms a stable hexamer precipitate in the neutral pH environment upon injection into subcutaneous tissue. The hexamer precipitate allows for a delay in the onset of action as well as a constant release of insulin over a 24-hour period with no pronounced peak.[2] As a result, glargine provides basal insulin action over the course of a given day. Because it is in an acid solution, glargine cannot be mixed with other forms of insulin because it would alter the absorption profiles of those insulins. In a comparison in patients with type 2 diabetes, the injection of bedtime insulin glargine resulted in a much lower frequency of nocturnal hypoglycemia but similar glycemic control and similar or less weight gain than bedtime NPH.[3] Moreover, the use of insulin glargine plus oral agents resulted in 56% fewer episodes of nocturnal hypoglycemia and significantly lower dinnertime plasma-glucose levels than NPH plus oral agents.[4]

***Insulin detemir:*** Also a recombinant human insulin analogue, insulin detemir has a 14-carbon fatty acid (myristic acid) covalently bound to lysine at position B29 and threonine at position B30 is omitted. Fatty acid acylation enhances detemir's affinity to albumin. Albumin binding enables detemir's protracted duration of effect via delayed absorption from the subcutaneous adipose tissue depot at the insulin injection site.[5] Detemir's duration of action is longer than that of NPH insulin, and its duration of action increases dose dependently from 5.7 hours at a low dose (0.1 units [U]/kg) to 23.2 hours at a high dose (1.6 U/kg).[6] However, detemir's duration of action in some cases is <24 hours. This is particularly so when the total daily insulin requirement is low (<0.1 U/kg/day) as may be the case in type 1 diabetes. For most type 2 diabetes patients, insulin detemir can be administered twice daily.

***NPH insulin:*** NPH or isophane insulin (Humulin® N, Novolin® N) is a crystalline suspension of insulin with protamine and zinc. NPH insulin's combined with protamine and low concentrations of zinc enhances its aggregation into dimers and hexamers after subcutaneous injection. A depot is formed after injection, and the insulin is released slowly, providing an intermediate-acting insulin with a slower onset of action and a longer duration of activity (ie, 12 to 16 hours) than regular insulin. NPH insulin's duration of action is variable; some patients rarely require only one NPH injection daily, whereas others require three or more injections daily. NPH insulin is equipotent to the other basal insulins, and it has variable absorption and peaks, both of which can predispose to hypoglycemia especially when a meal is delayed or food intake is curtailed. NPH insulin is now rarely used alone as basal insulin in type 2 patients unless given in a fixed combination (see Fixed-Combination Insulin below).

## Bolus Insulin

The term bolus insulin incorporates both prandial and correction doses of insulin. Bolus insulin is preferentially provided as one of the rapid-acting insulin analogues that are aspart (NovoLog®), glulisine (Apidra®), and lispro (Humalog®), or may be provided as short-acting regular insulin or inhaled insulin. Prandial or meal insulin refers to insulin that covers the postmeal glycemic excursion. An effort is made to match meal insulin doses to anticipated carbohydrate intake, which will be achieved either by a consistent carbohydrate meal plan or by carbohydrate counting, which is counting the number of carbohydrate grams consumed during a meal and calculating an appropriate dose of insulin to take with food.

Correction- or supplemental-dose insulin is used to treat hyperglycemia that occurs before or between meals despite the administration of routine daily doses of basal and prandial insulin, and is taken in addition to standing doses.

Bolus insulins can be categorized into rapid-acting insulin analogues (ie, aspart, glulisine, lispro), short-acting (regular) insulin, and inhaled insulin.

## Rapid-Acting Insulin

Rapid-acting insulin analogues are generally preferred as the bolus insulin of choice in intensive glycemic control regimens.[7,8] Their rapid time to onset of action allows injection immediately before meals, whereas short-acting (regular) insulin must be given 30 to 45 minutes before meals to optimally match the glycemic excursions after a meal.

Insulin lispro is recombinant deoxyribonucleic acid (DNA) combining Lys (B28) and Pro (B29) insulins. The effect of this amino acid rearrangement is to reduce the capacity of the insulin to self-aggregate in subcutaneous tissues, resulting in behavior that is similar to monomeric insulin and allowing more rapid absorption from the subcutaneous depot following injection. Given intravenously, the pharmacokinetic profiles of lispro and human regular insulin are similar. Insulin lispro was the first available rapid-acting insulin analogue that closely matches circulating insulin levels to the time course of the increase in plasma glucose seen after ingestion of a carbohydrate-rich meal.

Insulin aspart differs from human insulin by substitution of aspartic acid for proline at position B28. This substitution also leads to a more rapid onset and duration of action analogous to those seen with insulin lispro when compared with regular insulin.

Insulin glulisine is produced by recombinant DNA technology utilizing a nonpathogenic laboratory strain of *Escherichia coli* (K12). Insulin glulisine differs from human insulin in that asparagine at position B3 is replaced by lysine and the lysine in position B29 is replaced by glutamic acid.

### *Short-Acting (Regular) Insulin*

Short-acting (regular) insulin consists of zinc insulin crystals in monomeric form in a clear solution.[9] After subcutaneous injection, regular insulin tends to self-associate, first into dimers and then into hexamers, which must then dissociate before absorption because only monomers and dimers can be absorbed to any appreciable degree. This results in a 30-minute to 1-hour delay in the time it takes for regular insulin's onset following subcutaneous injection, which limits its flexibility in terms of convenience of time of administration in relationship to meals for the patient. Furthermore, because the peak glycemic response to a mixed meal is between 2 to 4 hours after ingestion, regular insulin may peak too late to allow targeted control of postprandial hyperglycemia. Finally, there is also a potential for hypoglycemia to develop as a late sequelae several hours after a meal has been absorbed because of regular insulin's longer duration of action, which often limits the ability of regular insulin to titrate to tight postprandial plasma glucose (PPG) goals.

### Inhaled Insulin

The US Food and Drug Administration (FDA) has approved an inhaled insulin (human [rDNA origin]) delivery system (Exubera®) for the management of type 1 and type 2 diabetes.[10,11] Exubera® insulin inhalation powder causes a rapid rise in serum insulin concentration (similar to what occurs after subcutaneous insulin aspart, glulisine, and lispro are injected, and faster than subcutaneous regular insulin). It has a slightly longer duration of action than rapid-acting insulin analogues.

In the Exubera® system, insulin inhalation powder is packaged in a foil blister pack that is inserted into an inhaler. A 1 mg capsule of Exubera® provides the equivalent of about 2.7 to 3 U of insulin, and the 3 mg capsule provides about 8 U. When the device is activated, the blister is pierced and the insulin powder is dispersed into a chamber that the patient then inhales through a mouthpiece.

The urge to cough is a problem with inhaled insulin. In one study, the incidence of coughing was 21%, compared with 4% to 8% for patients not using inhaled insulin. The use of inhaled insulin also causes a decrease in carbon monoxide diffusing capacity, although its effects on forced expiratory volume in 1 second ($FEV_1$), forced vital capacity (FVC), and total lung volume were not different compared with patients injecting subcutaneous insulin. Smoking may increase the effect of inhaled insulin; therefore, inhaled insulin is contraindicated in current or recent (ie, within the past 6 months) smokers, and in patients with asthma, chronic obstructive pulmonary disease (COPD), or other lung diseases.

## Table 7-2: Premixed Combination Insulins

| Premixed Insulin | Components |
|---|---|
| Humulin® 70/30, Novolin® 70/30 | 70% NPH/30% regular |
| Humulin® 50/50 | 50% NPH/50% regular |
| Humalog® Mix 50/50 | 50% lispro protamine/ 50% lispro |
| Humalog® Mix 75/25 | 75% lispro protamine/ 25% lispro |
| NovoLog® Mix 70/30 | 70% aspart protamine/ 30% aspart |

NPH=Neutral Protamine Hagedorn

### Fixed-Combination Insulin

Many patients with type 2 diabetes can use premixed preparations with reasonable effect. Premixtures increase the accuracy, effectiveness, and convenience of insulin dosing, which may improve compliance, long-term control, and outcome.[12]

A list of combination insulins is presented in Table 7-2. All combination insulins have a fixed percentage of an intermediate-acting insulin and a short- or rapid-acting insulin.

### Insulin Indications and Dosages

Insulin is usually prescribed to treat type 2 diabetes that cannot be properly controlled by diet, exercise, and weight loss. Insulin can be given to almost all patients regardless of stage of disease.[13] However, by convention, the principal indication for the use of insulin in type 2 diabetes is the failure of one and multiple oral agents, even when prescribed in combination, to maintain glycemic control. Insulin is also the treatment of choice to maintain glycemic control in many special circumstances, such as pregnancy, patients with ketonuria or ketonemia, patients in catabolic state (ie, very high plasma glucose with hyperglycemic symptoms and weight loss), and patients in the hospital.

Dosages must be tailored to the individual needs of each patient. During adolescent growth spurts, 0.8 to 1.2 U/kg/day is recommended, but for most children and adults, 0.5 to 1 U/kg/day has a near-maximal effect on plasma-glucose levels.[14] Of course, these formulas provide rough estimates, and specific insulin dosing should be tailored according to each patient, based on weight, glycemic control, and other factors (ie, nutrition, exercise). If the patient is prescribed a twice-daily premixed insulin, the dose is split into two thirds in the morning (ie, before breakfast) and one third in the evening (ie, before dinner). A patient could be prescribed a split regimen of basal and bolus insulins; the ideal regimen would be glargine at bedtime and rapid-acting insulin with meals. The total insulin dose is usually divided into 50% basal and 50% bolus (split into three times a day, if the patient eats three meals). The bolus dose is best given based on counting the carbohydrate content of the subsequent meal.

If a bedtime dose of glargine or detemir insulin is being added to oral hypoglycemic drug therapy, it is recommended to start at 10 to 12 U, which should be taken at 10 PM if the patient is testing his or her fasting plasma-glucose (FPG) level at 7 AM or 8 AM). FPG level should be measured every day. An increase of 2 to 6 U in the bedtime insulin dose should be made periodically (ie, every 3 to 7 days) until the patient's FPG is within goal.

## Exenatide

### *Background and Mechanism of Action*

Exenatide (Byetta®) belongs to the novel class of incretin mimetics because of its incretin-like action. Exenatide is a synthetic exendin-4 and is the first glucagon-like peptide-1

(GLP-1)-based therapy to be approved in the United States by the FDA for the treatment of type 2 diabetes in patients not sufficiently controlled with oral agents.

The two known incretins are the gastrointestinal (GI) hormones glucose-dependent insulinotropic peptide (GIP) and GLP-1, which stimulate insulin secretion after a meal. They are the reason why orally administered glucose evokes a greater insulin response than an intravenously administered glucose infusion calculated to lead to identical serum-glucose excursions. The difference in the insulin response is called the incretin effect.[15] The incretin effect is reduced or even absent in patients with type 2 diabetes.[16,17] Of the two incretins, GLP-1 has been the most widely studied.

Compared with other insulinotropic agents (eg, sulfonylureas), the insulinotropic effect of GLP-1 depends on the plasma's actual glucose concentration to provide the possibility of glucose normalization without the risk of hypoglycemic episodes. In addition to its glucose-lowering effects, GLP-1 has a variety of noninsulinotropic physiologic actions[18] that may be advantageous in type 2 diabetes therapy—it suppresses glucagon secretion from $\alpha$-cells and slows gastric emptying. Additionally, GLP-1 acts as a mediator of satiety in the hypothalamus, which decreases appetite, creating the potential for weight loss. When added to metformin-treated patients at 10 µg subcutaneously twice daily, after 30 weeks, exenatide lowered $HbA_{1c}$ by 0.78% and reduced weight an average of 2.8 kg compared to baseline.[19] Similarly, when added to patients on sulfonylurea, 10 µg twice daily of exenatide lowered $HbA_{1c}$ by 0.86% at 30 weeks, with a mean reduction of 1.6 kg body weight compared to baseline.

GLP-1 exhibits a short half-life of 1 to 2 minutes as the result of N-terminal degradation by the enzyme dipeptidyl peptidase IV (DPP-IV). Exendin-4, a long-acting potent agonist of the GLP-1 receptor, is a naturally occurring component of the saliva of the Gila monster (*Heloderma suspectum*), and shares 53% sequence identity with GLP-1. It is resistant to DPP-IV degradation[20] and, therefore, has a prolonged half-life.

### Indications and Dosages

Exenatide is used as a combination therapy with oral agents (ie, metformin, sulfonylureas, thiazolidinediones [TZDs] [Actos® (pioglitazone), Avandia® (rosiglitazone), Avandamet® (rosiglitazone/metformin)])[19,21,22] and is not approved for use as monotherapy or with insulin. Byetta® is available in prefilled syringes that hold a month's supply of either 5 or 10 μg doses, is administered subcutaneously twice daily immediately before or within 1 hour of morning and evening meals. The 5 μg dose is used the first month, then, if tolerated, can be increased to 10 μg.

### Side Effects and Warnings

Nausea is a common adverse effect of exenatide[20-22] but is generally mild to moderate in intensity and wanes with duration of therapy. Nausea can be reduced with dose titration. Mild-to-moderate hypoglycemic events occur only when exenatide is given in conjunction with a sulfonylurea; titrating the dose of sulfonylurea down to the smallest tablet size reduces hypoglycemia without substantially sacrificing efficacy.

Exenatide is not recommended for patients with gastroparesis, severe GI disease, or renal impairment (creatinine clearance [$C_{cr}$] <30 mL/min) due to frequent GI adverse effects. It can be safely used in patients with heart or liver disease.

Because of its effects on gastric emptying, exenatide may reduce the rate and extent of absorption of orally administered drugs. It should be used with caution in patients receiving medications that require rapid absorption from the GI tract. Medication administration 1 hour before the use of exenatide has been recommended when optimal drug absorption and peak levels are important to its overall therapeutic effect (ie, with antibiotics and/or oral contraceptives).

# Amylin and Pramlintide

## Background and Mechanism of Action

Amylin is a β-cell hormone that is co-located and co-secreted with insulin, playing a complementary role by regulating the rate of glucose secretion during the postprandial period. It does so through several mechanisms of action: slowing gastric emptying, suppressing inappropriate postprandial glucagon secretion, and regulating food intake.[23] Patients with type 1 diabetes and advanced type 2 diabetes have insulin and amylin deficiency; therefore, besides giving these patients insulin, also adding amylin could potentially benefit many of them through its mechanisms of action. Amylin has not been pursued as a pharmacologic preparation due to its low solubility and a propensity to aggregate. Pramlintide (Symlin®) is a synthetic, soluble, nonaggregating analogue of amylin with similar mechanisms of action that collectively regulate the secretion of glucose in the circulation following meals.

## Indications and Dosages

Pramlintide is only approved for use in patients who are also taking insulin. Pramlintide precipitates above a pH of 5.5 and must be injected separately from insulin at a different site.[24] The optimal timing for administration is immediately before a meal. Preprandial insulin dosages (including premixed insulin) should be reduced by 30% to 50%, and should subsequently be titrated upward to achieve euglycemia once the target pramlintide dosage is reached.

Pramlintide is currently only available in vials; the pen formulation will be available by the end of 2007. The recommended starting dosage for type 1 diabetes is 15 µg before each meal, with increases of 15 µg increments every 3 to 7 days, as tolerated, to a goal of 60 µg (or 10 U if administered in an insulin syringe). Persistent nausea should prompt backward titration until it is resolved.

The recommended initial dosage for type 2 diabetes is 60 μg, titrated upward, as tolerated, to 120 μg with each meal.

### Side Effects and Warnings

Mild-to-moderate nausea is the most commonly reported side effect and generally dissipates by the fourth week on pramlintide.[25] Nausea can be minimized by slow upward dose titration and is less common in patients with type 2 diabetes. Hypoglycemia can occur if mealtime insulin is not reduced appropriately after pramlintide is initiated. Pramlintide should not be administered to patients with severe hypoglycemia unawareness. Pramlintide should only be administered before meals that contain at least 250 calories or 30 g of carbohydrates. Patients may need to administer prandial insulin after meals until they become familiar with the degree of satiety and resulting reduction of carbohydrate intake that may occur.

Pramlintide slows gastric emptying and may delay the rate of absorption of oral medications. Patients with gastroparesis should not use pramlintide. Oral medications that require rapid absorption for effectiveness should be administered either 1 hour before or 2 hours after the injection of pramlintide.

## References

1.  Buse J: Combining insulin and oral agents. *Am J Med* 2000;108(suppl 6a):23S-32S.

2.  Lepore M, Pampanelli S, Fanelli C, et al: Pharmacokinetics and pharmacodynamics of subcutaneous injection of long-acting human insulin analogue glargine, NPH insulin, and ultralente human insulin and continuous subcutaneous infusion of insulin lispro. *Diabetes* 2000;49:2142-2148.

3.  Owens DR, Zinman B, Bolli GB: Insulins today and beyond. *Lancet* 2001;358:739-746; erratum *Lancet* 2001;358:1374.

4.  Yki-Jarvinen H: Combination therapies with insulin in type 2 diabetes. *Diabetes Care* 2001;24:758-767.

5. Havelund S, Plum A, Ribel U, et al: The mechanism of protraction of insulin detemir, a long-acting, acylated analog of human insulin. *Pharm Res* 2004;21:1498-1504.

6. Plank J, Bodenlenz M, Sinner F, et al: A double-blind, randomized, dose-response study investigating the pharmacodynamic and pharmacokinetic properties of the long-acting insulin analog detemir. *Diabetes Care* 2005;28:1107-1112.

7. Howey DC, Bowsher RR, Brunelle RL, et al: [Lys(B28), Pro(B29)]-human insulin. A rapidly absorbed analogue of human insulin. *Diabetes* 1994;43:396-402.

8. Hirsch IB: Insulin analogues. *N Engl J Med* 2005;352:174-183.

9. Plank J, Siebenhofer A, Berghold A, et al: Systematic review and meta-analysis of short-acting insulin analogues in patients with diabetes mellitus. *Arch Intern Med* 2005;165:1337-1344.

10. Hollander PA, Blonde L, Rowe R, et al: Efficacy and safety of inhaled insulin (exubera) compared with subcutaneous insulin therapy in patients with type 2 diabetes: results of a 6-month, randomized, comparative trial. *Diabetes Care* 2004;27:2356-2362.

11. Cefalu WT: Evolving strategies for insulin delivery and therapy. *Drugs* 2004;64:1149-1161.

12. Turner HE, Matthews DR: The use of fixed-mixture insulins in clinical practice. *Eur J Clin Pharmacol* 2000;56:19-25.

13. Evans A, Krentz AJ: Benefits and risks of transfer from oral agents to insulin in type 2 diabetes mellitus. *Drug Saf* 1999;21:7-22.

14. Berger M, Jorgens V, Muhlhauser I: Rationale for the use of insulin therapy alone as the pharmacological treatment of type 2 diabetes. *Diabetes Care* 1999;22(suppl 3):C71-C75.

15. Creutzfeldt W: The incretin concept today. *Diabetologia* 1979;16:75-85.

16. Creutzfeldt W: Entero-insular axis and diabetes mellitus. *Horm Metab Res Suppl* 1992;26:13-18.

17. Nauck MA, Heimesaat MM, Orskov C, et al: Preserved incretin activity of glucagon-like peptide 1 [7-36 amide] but not of synthetic human gastric inhibitory polypeptide in patients with type-2 diabetes mellitus. *J Clin Invest* 1993;91:301-307.

18. Parkes DG, Pittner R, Jodka C, et al: Insulinotropic actions of exendin-4 and glucagon-like peptide-1 in vivo and in vitro. *Metabolism* 2001;50:583-589.

19. DeFronzo RA, Ratner RE, Han J, et al: Effects of exenatide (exendin-4) on glycemic control and weight over 30 weeks in metformin-treated patients with type 2 diabetes. *Diabetes Care* 2005;28:1092-1100.

20. Gallwitz B: Therapies for the treatment of type 2 diabetes mellitus based on incretin action. *Minerva Endocrinol* 2006;31:133-147.

21. Buse JB, Henry RR, Han J, and Exenatide-113 Clinical Study Group, et al: Effects of exenatide (exendin-4) on glycemic control over 30 weeks in sulfonylurea-treated patients with type 2 diabetes. *Diabetes Care* 2004;27:2628-2635.

22. Zinman B, Hoogwerf BJ, Duran Garcia S, et al: The effect of adding exenatide to a thiazolidinedione in suboptimally controlled type 2 diabetes: a randomized trial. *Ann Intern Med* 2007;146: 477-485.

23. Singh-Franco D, Robles G, Gazze D: Pramlintide acetate injection for the treatment of type 1 and type 2 diabetes mellitus. *Clin Ther* 2007;29:535-562.

24. Schmitz O, Brock B, Rungby J: Amylin agonists: a novel approach in the treatment of diabetes. *Diabetes* 2004;53(suppl 3): S233-S238.

25. Hollander PA, Levy P, Fineman MS, et al: Pramlintide as an adjunct to insulin therapy improves long-term glycemic and weight control in patients with type 2 diabetes: a 1-year randomized controlled trial. *Diabetes Care* 2003;26:784-790.

7

## Chapter 8

# Successful Combination Therapy Strategies

The achievement of long-term normal glycemia in type 2 diabetes is difficult to accomplish with a single agent. After a successful initial response to oral therapy, patients fail to maintain target glycosylated hemoglobin $A_{1c}$ ($HbA_{1c}$) levels (<6.5% to 7%) at a rate of 5% to 10%/year. An analysis from the United Kingdom Prospective Diabetes Study (UKPDS) found that 50% of patients originally controlled with a single drug required the addition of a second drug after 3 years; at the end of 9 years, 75% of patients needed multiple therapies to achieve their target glycosylated $HbA_{1c}$ value.[1]

Among the factors that can contribute to worsening glycemic control are

- Decreased compliance with diet target goals,
- Decreased compliance with exercise regimen,
- Decreased compliance with medical regimen,
- Increased weight gain, and
- Progression of the underlying disease process, including insulin resistance and deficient insulin secretion, leading to the development of type 2 diabetes.

A 2006 consensus statement from the American Diabetes Association (ADA) and the European Association for the Study of Diabetes (EASD) proposes that metformin (Glucophage®, Glucophage® XR, Glumetza™) therapy (in the absence of contraindications) be initiated[2] concurrent with lifestyle modifications, at the time of diabetes diagnosis. This is because metformin often leads to modest weight reduction or weight stabilization, in contrast with most oral antidiabetic drugs.[3] In addition, obese patients in the UKPDS who were assigned initially to receive metformin rather than a sulfonylurea (glimepiride [Amaryl®], glyburide [DiaBeta®, Micronase®], micronized glyburide [Glynase® PresTab®] glipizide [Glucotrol®, Glucotrol XL®]), or insulin therapy had a decreased risk of the aggregate diabetes-related end point and all-cause mortality.[4] However, patients who are prescribed metformin eventually need another agent or additional treatment. Some patients also cannot take metformin because of heart failure, renal or hepatic insufficiency, or gastrointestinal (GI) issues. The different classes of antidiabetic drugs are reviewed in other chapters of this handbook. In this chapter, we review the most commonly used combination therapies.

## Combination Therapy With Oral Agents

Combination therapy with oral agents has several advantages. For many drugs, dosage and benefit are not directly proportional; therefore, half the maximum dosage produces more than half the maximum therapeutic effect, with fewer side effects. Thus, when agents are combined, lower doses of each can be used to enhance outcomes and, often, to reduce costs. Different combinations can be used: metformin and a secretagogue (ie, a sulfonylurea or a meglitinide); metformin and a thiazolidinedione (TZD) (Actos® [pioglitazone], Avandia® [rosiglitazone], Avandamet® [rosiglitazone/metformin]); a secretagogue plus a TZD; sitagliptin (Januvia™) plus metformin (Janumet™); sitagliptin plus a TZD; and triple therapy, such as metformin, a sulfonylurea, and a TZD. Each of these combinations has been studied and showed an additive hypoglycemic effect when adding a second agent. α-Glucosidase inhibitors are not commonly used

## Table 8-1: Fixed Combinations of Oral Agents

| Oral Agent | Components |
|---|---|
| Metaglip™ | Glipizide (Glucotrol®, Glucotrol XL®)/metformin (Glucophage®, Glucophage® XR, Glumetza™) |
| Glucovance® | Glyburide (DiaBeta®, Micronase®)/metformin |
| Avandamet® | Rosiglitazone (Avandia®)/metformin |
| ACTO*plus* met® | Pioglitazone (Actos®)/metformin |
| Avandaryl™ | Rosiglitazone/glimepiride (Amaryl®) |
| Duetact™ | Pioglitazone (Actos®)/glimepiride |
| Janumet™ | Sitagliptin (Januvia™)/metformin |

in the United States because of their poorer tolerance and lower efficacy.

Although triple oral agent therapy is a reasonable approach, few data are available on optimal combinations, dosages, and outcomes. Before proceeding with triple-oral-agent therapy, careful consideration of its cost relative to that of insulin therapy is required. Less challenging insulin delivery systems and a new class of parenteral therapy (ie, incretin mimetics) may make triple-oral-agent therapy less attractive.

**Dosage Form (mg)**

2.5/250, 2.5/500, 5/500

1.25/250, 2.5/500, 5/500

2/500, 4/500, 2/1,000, 4/1,000

15/500, 15/850

4/1, 4/2, 4/4, 8/2, 8/4

30/2, 30/4

50/500, 50/1,000

Selecting a combination therapy depends on the following factors:
- Contraindications to using a particular drug or potential for problems by using a certain drug (ie, renal insufficiency, heart failure, hepatic insufficiency related to the use of metformin, heart failure related to the use of TZDs);
- Risks of hypoglycemia from insulin secretagogues in selected patients (eg, the elderly, patients suffering from renal failure)—in patients at risk for hypoglycemia,

consideration should be given to drugs that do not cause hypoglycemia, such as metformin, TZDs, and sitagliptin, assuming there are no other contraindications to using those drugs;

• Weight gain issues (ie, the use of TZDs).

More in-depth discussions of selected agents are featured in other chapters in this handbook. Table 8-1 summarizes the fixed combinations of oral agents that are currently available.

## Combination Therapy
## With Oral Agents and Insulin

Insulin is a reasonable choice for initial therapy in patients who present with symptomatic or poorly controlled diabetes (HbA$_{1c}$ ≥10%), and it is the preferred second-line medication for patients with HbA$_{1c}$ >8.5% to 9% or with symptoms of hyperglycemia who are already being treated with metformin.

Insulin and oral agents may be combined to improve the glycemic control exerted by significant, but ineffective, doses of either, or to reduce the dose or eliminate the need for the original therapy (most commonly insulin) while reducing side effects, or using properties of the other agent.[5-7] If large doses of insulin do not produce adequate glycemic control, the addition of an oral agent to insulin therapy may be considered. This combination therapy improves glycemic control and reduces the required insulin dosage and residual weight gain associated with insulin therapy. In particular, metformin may help offset the weight gain associated with insulin therapy. No study has reported worse glycemic control with combination therapy than on insulin alone, and randomized, prospective clinical trial data support combining insulin therapy with metformin and TZDs for enhanced glycemic control. Modest improvement in glycemic control has been documented through the combination of insulin therapy with sulfonylureas.

It should be noted that the combination of insulin with either rosiglitazone or pioglitazone has been associated with an increased incidence of fluid overload and should be avoided in patients with heart failure.

## Other Combination Therapies
### *Exenatide and Oral Agents*

As discussed in Chapter 6, exenatide (Byetta®) can be combined with oral agents.[9-11] Even though it needs to be injected, exenatide offers the possibility of weight loss and can be a preferred second-line agent after metformin.

### *Pramlintide and Insulin*

As discussed in Chapter 7, pramlintide (Symlin®) can be combined with insulin, improving glycemic control and inducing weight loss.[12]

## Recommendations

A 2006 consensus statement from the ADA and the EASD proposed that metformin therapy (in the absence of contraindications) be initiated, concurrent with lifestyle modifications, at the time of diabetes diagnosis.[2] Although diet, weight loss, and regular exercise can markedly improve glucose metabolism, compliance with these interventions is not sustained in most patients.

Metformin therapy should be initiated in most patients at the time of diabetes diagnosis, in the absence of specific contraindications, and with a consultation for lifestyle intervention. The dose of metformin should be titrated to its maximally effective dose (2,000 mg daily) as tolerated. Metformin should not be given to the elderly (>80 years) unless renal sufficiency is proven with a direct measure of glomerular filtration rate (GFR), or to patients who have renal or hepatic insufficiency or who have had heart failure. Another agent should be prescribed in these cases.

Patients who are underweight (ie, patients who may have type 1 diabetes), are losing weight, and are symptomatic from hyperglycemia, or are ketotic should be started on insulin, regardless of age. Insulin may be considered initial therapy for patients with type 2 diabetes presenting with very high $HbA_{1c}$ >10% to 11%.

If adequate control is not achieved ($HbA_{1c}$ remains >6.5% to 7%), another medication should be added within 3 to 6 months after lifestyle intervention and the addition of metformin. It should be anticipated that most patients will require early combination therapy to achieve these glycemic goals based on the older UKPDS data as well as analysis of more recent publications.[1,2,12] From the many possible choices of second-line agents, the clinician must rely on the available safety and efficacy data. Recently, more clinical trials have supported the use of various combination therapies of antidiabetic agents, as early therapy or even in drug-naive subjects.

The most common oral agents used in early combination with metformin include sulfonylureas, TZDs, and more recently, sitagliptin. Injectable agents (exenatide or insulin) may also be added to metformin therapy for early combined treatment. Each of these approaches uses a different mechanism of drug action, and, consequently, they exhibit additive or synergistic effects in glucose lowering. It should be noted that unanticipated side effects can accompany the clinical use of any of these agents, even in combination.

The best strategy is to minimize adverse side effects by employing submaximal doses of drugs in combination, especially those with predictable issues, ie, hypoglycemia with sulfonylureas, weight gain and peripheral edema with TZDs, GI effects of high doses of metformin. The insulin secretion enhancers are effective in glucose lowering, but hypoglycemia is common, especially when these drugs are used aggressively early in the course of the disease. For example, one trial of initial combination therapy with glyburide/metformin (Glucovance®), 72% of patients with a mean $HbA_{1c}$ of 8.2% achieved a goal $HbA_{1c}$ of <7%, but episodes of hypoglycemia were reported in 38%.[13] In contrast, the initial combination of rosiglitazone/metformin (Avandamet®) therapy reportedly enabled 77% of subjects starting with a mean $HbA_{1c}$ of 8.9% to achieve $HbA_{1c}$ at 32 weeks without significant hypoglycemia.[14] Using metformin with rosiglitazone abrogated weight gain anticipated with the TZD, although the rosiglitazone-treated subjects experienced more peripheral edema. A recent study using initial treatment with sitagliptin/metformin (Janumet™) showed the combination to be well tolerated and highly effective with 66% of subjects starting with a mean $HbA_{1c}$ of 8.8% achieving $HbA_{1c}$ <7% at 24 weeks.[15]

Additional factors to consider in choosing medications for combination therapy include:

- Metformin can abrogate the weight gain observed with sulfonylureas, TZDs, or insulin, but the GI side effects of metformin are usually dose related.
- Exenatide added early may benefit patients that need to lose weight, unless they refuse the twice-daily injection regimen or experience GI intolerance to the drug.
- Sitagliptin is a good choice for a second agent since it is well tolerated and performs well for glycemic lowering in combination; however, unlike exenatide, weight loss has not been observed with sitagliptin.
- Insulin (as a basal, premixed, or split regimen) can be used at any time; however, starting insulin injections necessitates overcoming the psychological barriers to insulin as well as concerns about weight gain and hypoglycemia.

Adjustments in therapy should not be made more frequently than every 3 months, based on the $HbA_{1c}$ result, aiming for levels as close to the nondiabetic range as possible, while avoiding weight gain, hypoglycemia and GI side effects whenever possible.

# References

1.   Turner RC, Cull CA, Frighi V, et al: Glycemic control with diet, sulfonylurea, metformin, or insulin in patients with type 2 diabetes. Progressive requirement for multiple therapies (UKPDS 49). UK Prospective Diabetes Study (UKPDS) Group. *JAMA* 1999;281: 2005-2012.

2.   Nathan DM, Buse JB, Davidson MB, et al: Management of hyperglycemia in type 2 diabetes: A consensus algorithm for the initiation and adjustment of therapy: a consensus statement from the American Diabetes Association and the European Association for the Study of Diabetes. *Diabetes Care* 2006;29:1963-1972.

3.   United Kingdom Prospective Diabetes Study (UKPDS). 13: Relative efficacy of randomly allocated diet, sulfonylureas, insulin, or metformin in patients with newly diagnosed non-insulin-dependent diabetes followed for three years. *BMJ* 1995;310:83-88.

4.   Effect of intensive blood-glucose control with metformin on complications in overweight patients with type 2 diabetes (UKPDS 34). UK Prospective Diabetes Study (UKPDS) Group. *Lancet* 1998;352:854-865.

5.   Buse J: Combining insulin and oral agents. *Am J Med* 2000; 108(suppl 6a):23S-32S.

6.   Buse JB: The use of insulin alone and in combination with oral agents in type 2 diabetes. *Prim Care* 1999;26:931-950.

7.   Yki-Jarvinen H: Combination therapies with insulin in type 2 diabetes. *Diabetes Care* 2001;24:758-767.

8.   DeFronzo RA, Ratner RE, Han J, et al: Effects of exenatide (exendin-4) on glycemic control and weight over 30 weeks in metformin-treated patients with type 2 diabetes. *Diabetes Care* 2005;28:1092-1100.

9.   Buse JB, Henry RR, Han J, et al: Effects of exenatide (exendin-4) on glycemic control over 30 weeks in sulfonylurea-treated patients with type 2 diabetes. *Diabetes Care* 2004;27:2628-2635.

10.   Zinman B, Hoogwerf BJ, Duran Garcia S, et al: The effect of adding exenatide to a thiazolidinedione in suboptimally controlled type 2 diabetes: a randomized trial. *Ann Intern Med* 2007;146:477-485.

11.   Schmitz O, Brock B, Rungby J: Amylin agonists: a novel approach in the treatment of diabetes. *Diabetes* 2004;53(suppl 3): S233-S238.

12.   Goldstein BJ: Clinical translation of "a diabetes outcome progression trial": ADOPT appropriate combination oral therapies in type 2 diabetes. *J Clin Endocrinol Metab* 2007;92:1226-1228.

13.   Garber AJ, Larsen J, Schneider SH, et al: Simultaneous glyburide/metformin therapy is superior to component monotherapy as an initial pharmacological treatment for type 2 diabetes. *Diabetes Obes Metab* 2002;4:201-208.

14.   Rosenstock J, Rood J, Cobitz A, et al:  Initial treatment with rosiglitazone/metformin fixed-dose combination therapy compared with monotherapy with either rosiglitazone or metformin in patients with uncontrolled type 2 diabetes. *Diabetes Obes Metab* 2006;8: 650-660.

15.   Goldstein BJ, Feinglos MN, Lunceford JK, et al, for the Sitagliptin 036 Study Group: Effect of initial combination therapy with sitagliptin, a dipeptidyl peptidase-4 inhibitor, and metformin on glycemic control in patients with type 2 diabetes. *Diabetes Care* 2007;30:1979-1987.

8

*Chapter* **9**

# Macrovascular Complications — Prevention and Management

Ａll of the metabolic abnormalities of diabetes, including dyslipidemia, hypertension, hypercoagulability, hyperglycemia, and hyperinsulinemia, contribute to cardiovascular disease (CVD), and therefore, all are appropriate therapeutic targets. The presence of more than one risk factor exponentially increases CVD risk.[1] This finding, coupled with the heavy burden of CVD in patients with type 2 diabetes, has prompted the Joint National Committee on Prevention, Detection, Evaluation, and Treatment of High Blood Pressure (JNC 7), the American Diabetes Association (ADA), and the National Cholesterol Education Program (NCEP) to recommend aggressive, multifactorial risk factor modification in these patients. In the Steno-2 study, this approach reduced the combined risk of death, nonfatal myocardial infarction (MI) or stroke, revascularization, and amputation by 50% in patients with type 2 diabetes who were at particularly high CVD risk because of associated microalbuminuria.[2]

However, some CVD risk factors associated with diabetes increase risk more than others. For instance, the United Kingdom Prospective Diabetes Study (UKPDS) showed the most important MI risk factor to be elevated low-density lipoprotein cholesterol (LDL-C) level, followed by elevated diastolic blood pressure, cigarette smoking, a low high-density lipoprotein cholesterol (HDL-C) level, and a high level of glycosylated hemoglobin $A_{1c}$ ($HbA_{1c}$).[3] Although multifactorial intervention has been proven to reduce the burden of CVD in patients with type 2 diabetes, early recognition and aggressive management of the major CVD risk factors are the main priorities in the delivery of diabetes care. The importance of these risk factors may vary for each patient. These include therapeutic lifestyle changes with accompanying weight loss, smoking cessation, appropriate antiplatelet agents (5-aminosalicylic acid [5-ASA], at a dose of 81 mg), together with reducing glucose, blood pressure, and lipids to appropriate levels.

## Hypertension

Hypertension is defined by the JNC 7[1] as blood pressure ≥130/80 mm Hg. It affects up to 70% of patients with type 2 diabetes and is twice as prevalent in diabetics as in nondiabetics.[4] Hypertension accounts for 30% to 70% of diabetic complications and worsens CVD, renal disease, peripheral vascular disease (PVD), stroke, and diabetic retinopathy.[4] Furthermore, hypertension accelerates diabetic cardiomyopathy, resulting in left-ventricular hypertrophy (LVH) and ultimately heart failure. Serious cardiovascular events are two or three times as likely to occur in diabetic hypertensive patients as in those with either diabetes or hypertension alone. In type 2 diabetic patients, dyslipidemia and endothelial abnormalities add to the increased cardiovascular risk from hypertension.[5] End-stage renal disease (ESRD) is five to six times more likely to develop in hypertensive patients with diabetes than in hypertensive patients without diabetes. Hypertension increases diabetic mortality fourfold to fivefold because of its contribution to renal disease and CVD.

### Treatment Rationale and Goals

Solid clinical trial data have established the effectiveness of aggressive treatment of hypertension in reducing the diabetic vascular complication rate. In the UKPDS, every 10 mm Hg decrease in mean systolic blood pressure reduced risk by 12% for any diabetic complication, 15% for diabetes-related death, 11% for MI, and 13% for microvascular complications, and no risk threshold was found for any end point studied.[2]

The Hypertension Optimal Treatment (HOT) trial revealed that reaching a diastolic blood-pressure goal of 80 mm Hg resulted in 51% fewer cardiovascular events than reaching a goal of 90 mm Hg, supporting the importance of targeting lower blood pressures.[6] Elevated systolic blood pressure may contribute more to cardiovascular risk than elevated diastolic blood pressure.

## Angiotensin-converting Enzyme Inhibitors

*Indications:* Angiotensin-converting enzyme (ACE) inhibitors, either alone or in conjunction with a thiazide diuretic, are indicated for initial therapy of hypertension in the insulin-resistant individual. Both the Heart Outcomes Prevention the Evaluation (HOPE) trial (ramipril [Altace®] 10 mg) and the European Trial on the Reduction of Cardiac Events with Perindopril in Stable Coronary Artery Disease (EUROPA) (perindopril [Aceon®] 8 mg) lend support to the valuable cardioprotective properties of these two agents.[7,8]

*Adverse effects:* Although generally well tolerated, ACE inhibitors can cause cough in as many as 15% of patients, more commonly women, because they elevate bradykinin levels. Patients with renal dysfunction or who are receiving potassium-sparing diuretics, β-blockers, or nonsteroidal anti-inflammatory drugs (NSAIDs) may get hyperkalemia during ACE inhibitor therapy, although it is uncommon with serum creatinine levels of ≤2.5 mg/dL. Angioedema is a rare, serious ACE inhibitor side effect. Overall, however, ACE inhibitors are well tolerated.

## Angiotensin II Receptor Blockers

Angiotensin II receptor blockers (ARBs) have effects similar to those of ACE inhibitors, and recent trials (the

Irbesartan Diabetic Nephropathy Trial [IDNT],[9] Reduction of Endpoints in Non-Insulin-Dependent Diabetes Mellitus with the Angiotensin Antagonist Losartan [RENAAL] Study,[10] Losartan Intervention for Endpoint Reduction in Hypertension [LIFE] study,[11] and Valsartan Heart Failure Trial [ValHEFT])[12] suggest that ARBs are renoprotective and cardioprotective.[16,20-22] They also do not have the side effects of ACE inhibitors, particularly cough, and are often useful in patients who cannot tolerate ACE inhibitors because of cough.

*Adverse effects:* ARBs are remarkably safe. Hyperkalemia, short-term initial increases in serum creatinine level, and hematologic adverse effects have been extremely rare in clinical studies.

### α-Adrenergic Receptor Antagonists

*Adverse effects:* In the Antihypertensive and Lipid-Lowering Treatment to Prevent Heart Attack Trial (ALLHAT), doxazosin (Cardura®, Cardura® XL) was associated with a 25% higher risk of major cardiovascular events, defined as heart failure, stroke, angina, and coronary revascularizations, when compared with that for the diuretic chlorthalidone (Thalitone®). This statistically significant finding suggested that, despite its equivalent hypotensive effect, doxazosin is inferior to chlorthalidone as first-line therapy.[13] In addition, this finding raised the question of whether doxazosin should be used as add-on therapy. However, the higher cardiovascular risk found in ALLHAT was attributed to a doubling in risk of additional treatment or hospitalization for heart failure associated with doxazosin over that associated with chlorthalidone. Moreover, the mean baseline systolic blood pressure in the doxazosin group was 3 mm Hg higher than that in the chlorthalidone group, which, in the high-risk patients studied, could explain some of the difference in heart failure rates. Because of these limitations, additional data are needed on which to base decisions on α-blocker use for diabetic hypertension, particularly as add-on therapy. However, it appears prudent to reserve α-blockers for use as add-on drugs until clinical trial data can support a more prominent role for them.

***Contraindications and precautions:*** Because the first dose of α-blockers may cause syncope, therapy should always be initiated with a low dose, and patients should be advised to avoid situations in which injury could occur during syncope. Dose should be titrated slowly, and additional antihypertensives should be added with caution.

### β-Adrenergic Receptor Antagonists

***Adverse effects:*** By directly inhibiting pancreatic insulin release and decreasing serum insulin levels, β-blockers can worsen glucose tolerance.[14] As a class, these agents and diuretics pose a high risk for development of new-onset diabetes.[14] For these reasons, they should no longer be used as initial therapy in the uncomplicated patient with insulin resistance.

Combined α- and β-blockers such as carvedilol (Coreg®) have been shown to have potential anti-oxidant effects and thus potential insulin-sensitizing effects (Glycemic Effects in Diabetes Mellitus: Carvedilol-Metoprolol Comparison in Hypertensives [GEMINI] trial)[15] and thus are useful as second-line therapy to renin-angiotensin system (RAS) inhibitors. Carvedilol is now available in a once-daily, extended dosing formulation, Coreg CR™, which offers the advantage of increased patient compliance.

### Calcium-channel Blockers

The second most widely used antihypertensives, calcium-channel blockers (CCBs) are heterogeneous. Most CCBs are dihydropyridine derivatives, which do not decrease heart rate. In contrast, the nondihydropyridines do. All CCBs are potent vasodilators.

***Adverse effects:*** CCBs generally have no adverse effects on lipid profile or insulin sensitivity. Some of the most common adverse effects of CCB therapy in diabetic hypertensive patients include edema, headache, cough, and gastrointestinal (GI) tract disease.[16]

**Diuretics**

Diuretics not only lower blood pressure effectively but also reduce cardiovascular morbidity and mortality when used as monotherapy or in combination therapy, and their ability to provide these benefits in diabetic patients with systolic hypertension has been proven. In a large cohort of elderly diabetic patients with isolated systolic hypertension studied for 5 years by the Systolic Hypertension in the Elderly Program (SHEP), low-dose chlorthalidone-based treatment lowered blood pressure, prevented major cardiovascular events, and produced few adverse effects relative to placebo treatment.[17] Although the relative treatment benefit in patients with diabetes was similar to that in individuals without diabetes, the absolute benefit in terms of number of patients needed to treat to prevent one cardiovascular complication was lower in diabetic patients than in nondiabetic individuals. These results also refuted the notion that diuretics should be avoided in diabetic patients because they increase plasma-glucose levels. More recently, ALLHAT found chlorthalidone to be superior to amlodipine (Norvasc®) and lisinopril (Prinivil®, Zestril®) in reducing systolic blood pressure and in preventing heart failure. Chlorthalidone was also found to be superior to lisinopril in preventing stroke. As a result, the ALLHAT investigators recommended that thiazides be used as initial antihypertensive therapy in patients with hypertension and at least one other coronary artery disease (CAD) risk factor.[18]

*Adverse effects:* Diuretics may cause hypovolemia and electrolyte imbalance. Although diuretics are recommended for hypertensive diabetic patients, no consensus exists regarding their use in clinical practice. Many physicians do not prescribe thiazides because they may alter carbohydrate metabolism, increase insulin resistance, and promote hyperinsulinemia and dyslipidemia.

## Combination Therapy

Because hypertension is a multifactorial disease, interrupting a single contributory physiologic pathway is frequently insufficient to reach target blood pressure. Combining agents from different drug classes that affect different physiologic pathways may be required for adequate control.[19] Furthermore, adding a second antihypertensive agent is recommended if target blood pressure cannot be achieved with a single agent, and many, if not most, type 2 diabetic patients require combination therapy. For example, >65% of micro- or macroalbuminuric diabetic hypertensive patients studied in a review of clinical trials needed at least two antihypertensive agents to attain the current recommended target of 130/85 mm Hg. In the UKPDS, almost one third of patients (29%) required at least three antihypertensive agents to achieve an average blood pressure of 144/82 mm Hg, which, by current standards, would be considered high.[20] In the HOT trial, 73% of patients required about 2.7 different antihypertensive agents to reach a diastolic blood pressure of <80 mm Hg. Diabetic patients with renal insufficiency often require moderate-to-high doses of three different antihypertensives to reach lower blood-pressure targets. Thus, for most diabetic patients, reaching goals with monotherapy is challenging, particularly because fear of increased side effects and patient resistance make many clinicians reluctant to titrate the dose or change agents. Nevertheless, the most important factor in decreasing their high incidence of CAD may be aggressive early hypertension control, and one of the most important factors in slowing renal disease progression in patients with type 2 diabetes is the level of arterial pressure reduction, particularly systolic blood pressure. Using low-dose combination antihypertensive therapy either as first-line treatment or early in the disease course can meet many of these challenges, and it has been recommended as an alternative to standard first-line monotherapy in reducing hypertension. Low-dose combinations are more effective than monotherapy because of the additive and sometimes even synergistic hypotensive effects of these complementary agents.

## Dyslipidemia

In animal models, hypertension alone does not cause atherosclerosis when cholesterol levels are low. Human populations with a high incidence of hypertension but low cholesterol levels also have a relatively low incidence of atherosclerotic complications. These findings suggest that the atherogenic changes in endothelium and vascular smooth muscle promoted by hypertension do not themselves lead to atherosclerotic fatty streaks and plaque. For atherosclerosis to develop, LDL-C or very-low-density lipoprotein cholesterol (VLDL-C) levels must be elevated as well as blood pressure. Thus, although blood-pressure control is important, the antihypertensive agents used to achieve it should not promote dyslipidemia.[21]

### *Treatment Goals*

The National Cholesterol Education Program Adult Treatment Panel III (NCEP-ATP III) defined optimal plasma-lipid levels for adults with diabetes to be <200 mg/dL of total cholesterol, <100 mg/dL of LDL-C (with optional goal of <70 mg/dL), >45 mg/dL of HDL-C in men and 55 mg/dL in women, and <200 mg/dL triglycerides (Tgs).[22] Because patients with type 2 diabetes not only have a risk of CHD events about three times that of nondiabetic individuals but also have an increased risk of mortality from a first MI, these recommended lipid levels are the same as those for nondiabetic patients with CVD.

### *Lipid-lowering Agent Monotherapy*

### HMG-CoA Reductase Inhibitors (Statins)

The 3-hydroxy-3-methylglutaryl coenzyme A (HMG-CoA) reductase inhibitors, commonly known as statins, are the most effective agents for lowering LDL-C patients with type 2 diabetes.[23] In addition, statins can beneficially alter LDL-C subfraction profiles and significantly reduce Tg levels.

*Indications:* Statin therapy should be considered for all patients who are at increased risk for atherosclerosis-related events because of their LDL-C level and/or the additional cardiovascular risk posed by type 2 diabetes.

*Mechanism of action:* Statins act in the liver to inhibit HMG-CoA reductase, the rate-limiting enzyme in cholesterol synthesis.

*Effectiveness:* Statins typically reduce LDL-C by 30% to 60%, depending on potency of individual statin and statin dose. Statin dose may need to be titrated in response to the level of LDL-C reduction obtained with initial therapy and adjusted after 4 to 6 weeks.[23] Statins may increase HDL-C levels by 5% to 10%.

*Adverse effects:* All of the available statins are relatively well tolerated. The most commonly reported adverse effect of statins is minor GI disturbance and/or myalgic 'aches and pains' in absence of full-blown clinical myositis. Less common but more serious side effects include frank myositis, rhabdomyolysis, and elevated liver enzyme levels, which appear to be dose dependent.[24] Transient asymptomatic increases in hepatic transaminase levels have been reported in about 1% of patients receiving statin therapy. An increase of aspartate aminotransferase (AST) or alanine aminotransferase (ALT) above three times the upper limit of normal indicates that the dose must be reduced or treatment halted. Significant hepatic dysfunction is exceptionally rare with statins.

*Drug interactions:* Proximal myopathy and rhabdomyolysis are more common when statins are combined with fibrates, nicotinic acid (niacin), or cyclosporine (Gengraf®, Neoral®, Sandimmune®),[24] which impairs statin metabolism. Treatment with azole antifungal agents, erythromycin, clarithromycin (Biaxin®, Biaxin® XL), human immunodeficiency virus (HIV) protease inhibitors, nefazodone, or verapamil (Calan®, Covera-HS®, Isoptin® SR, Verelan®) can increase the risk of myopathy in patients receiving statin therapy, as can consuming large amounts of grapefruit juice. Patients taking some statins and coumarin anticoagulants have experienced bleeding and increased clotting times. As a result, patients taking these medications should have their blood coagulation profile measured before statin therapy is initiated and should be monitored regularly thereafter.

*Contraindications and precautions:* Statin therapy is contraindicated in pregnant patients and in patients with cholestasis, and should be used with caution in patients with liver dysfunction. Statin therapy should be avoided or discontinued if a pregnancy is planned and should be stopped when pregnancy is discovered and not resumed until breast feeding is completed. Pediatric use of statins is not recommended.[17]

### Fibrates

Gemfibrozil (Lopid®), and micronized fenofibrate (TriCor®) are the typical drugs in this class that are now approved for prescription use in the United States. As a class, fibrates are most effective in reducing plasma concentrations of Tg-rich lipoproteins such as VLDL and chylomicrons. They generally decrease Tg levels and increase HDL-C levels more than statins.[25]

Evidence that fibrate therapy may reduce the risk of cardiovascular events was supplied by the Helsinki Heart study, which included 135 patients with diabetes. In this primary prevention study, the 5-year incidence of major CHD events in diabetic patients without CHD who were treated with gemfibrozil was reduced by 68% vs the placebo-treated group. However, this difference did not reach statistical significance because of the small numbers of patients in the analysis of the subgroup with diabetes.[26] The utility of gemfibrozil in secondary CHD event prevention was also demonstrated in the Veterans Affairs Cooperative Studies Program HDL-cholesterol Intervention Trial (VA-HIT), in which 627 patients (25%), had diabetes. In this study, the cardiovascular event rate was reduced by 24% in gemfibrozil-treated patients with type 2 diabetes vs the placebo-treated group.[27] Finally, some doubt was cast on the beneficial cardiovascular outcomes in diabetics using fenofibrate (Lipofen™, TriCor®, Triglide™) in the recent Fenofibrate Intervention and Event Lowering in Diabetes (FIELD) trial.[28]

*Adverse effects:* Fibrates are generally well tolerated. The most common adverse effects are GI disturbances (ie, nausea, dyspepsia, diarrhea, abdominal pain.)

*Drug interactions:* Patients taking some fibrates and coumarin anticoagulants have experienced bleeding and increased clotting times; therefore, the dosage of anticoagulant should be decreased in these patients to keep prothrombin time (PT) at optimal levels, and frequent assessment of PT is recommended until this laboratory value stabilizes. Concomitant treatment with statins and fibrates, particularly gemfibrozil and fenofibrate, should be avoided unless the benefit is likely to outweigh the increased risk of diabetic myopathy. Interactions between fibrates, which are primarily excreted by the kidneys, and potentially nephrotoxic drugs, such as cyclosporine, may also pose problems. As a result, the benefits of using fibrates with potentially nephrotoxic immunosuppressants should be weighed against the risks, and the lowest effective doses should be used.

*Contraindications and precautions:* Results of animal studies showed fibrates to be embryocidal and teratogenic at high doses. Fibrates should, therefore, avoided during pregnancy.

## Nicotinic Acid

The hypolipidemic effects of nicotinic acid have been recognized for more than 40 years, and this agent has been used widely to treat hypercholesterolemia and combined hyperlipidemia[17] because of its excellent lipid-lowering properties. It is the most effective available agent for elevating HDL-C levels, and it decreases Tgs, LDL-C, and even lipoprotein(a) [LP(a)] levels.[1] Nicotinic acid is available in immediate-release or crystalline and sustained-release

(Niaspan®) forms. Nicotinic acid decreases insulin sensitivity and may therefore worsen glycemic control.

*Indications:* In patients with type 2 diabetes, nicotinic acid is typically used as a second-line agent in high-risk patients. Because nicotinic acid therapy can cause hyperglycemia, it may be particularly inappropriate for patients whose plasma-glucose levels are poorly controlled.[25]

*Effectiveness:* The largest reductions were seen in patients with the highest baseline levels of these lipids. In addition, HDL-C levels increased by 32%. The positive correlation between reductions in LDL-C and LP(a) concentrations observed in this study further indicates that nicotinic acid reduces the level of LP(a) through a reduction in LP(a) synthesis.

*Adverse effects:* The most common adverse effect of nicotinic acid is cutaneous flushing, which can be minimized by initiating therapy at low doses, slowly titrating the dose, and instructing the patient to take the drug with meals. Other side effects include paresthesias, abdominal discomfort, stomachaches, pruritus, dry skin, nausea, hepatitis, and, rarely, blurred vision. Flushing and paresthesias can be minimized by ingesting aspirin or NSAIDs 30 minutes before taking nicotinic acid.[4]

*Drug interactions:* Nicotinic acid potentiates the effects of antihypertensive agents, and concomitant administration of these medications may require adjustment of their dosage.

*Contraindications and precautions:* Because it may worsen hyperglycemia, nicotinic acid therapy is usually contraindicated in patients with type 2 diabetes. Nicotinic acid is also contraindicated in patients with a history of hyperuricemia or gout, peptic ulcer disease, or liver dysfunction because it may worsen these conditions. As a result, plasma glucose, uric acid, and hepatic enzyme levels should be monitored regularly in patients with type 2 diabetes who are receiving nicotinic acid therapy. An increase in hepatic enzyme levels to more than three times the upper limit of normal should trigger immediate discontinuation of nicotinic acid therapy.

Timed-release nicotinic acid may be hepatotoxic at dosages that exceed 2 g daily.

## Ezetimibe

Ezetimibe (Zetia®) is a new type of cholesterol-lowering agent that selectively reduces the absorption of cholesterol by >50%.

*Indications:* Ezetimibe is indicated as monotherapy and in combination with a statin for therapy of primary hypercholesterolemia to reduce total cholesterol and LDL-C.

*Mechanism of action:* Ezetimibe acts in the brush border of the small intestine to inhibit cholesterol transport across the intestinal wall. It is primarily metabolized by the small intestine and liver by glucuronidation, and excreted through the urine and bile. Its plasma half-life is approximately 22 hours. It can be administered with or without food.

*Effectiveness:* Alone or in combination with a statin, ezetimibe lowers total cholesterol, LDL-C, apolipoprotein B, and Tgs, and raises HDL-C. Its maximal effect is achieved within 2 weeks of initiation of therapy. Approximately 18% reduction in LDL-C can be significantly improved by synergizing with a statin.[29]

*Adverse effects:* Adverse effects that were reported in clinical trials with a significantly higher incidence than placebo included back pain and arthralgia in monotherapy, and back pain and abdominal pain in combination with a statin.

### Combination Lipid-lowering Agent Therapy

Combination therapy with two or sometimes three lipid-lowering agents is appropriate for adults with severe hypercholesterolemia or combined hyperlipidemia. Combination therapy with low doses of drugs with complementary mechanisms of action may be safer and better tolerated than high doses of a single agent and, therefore, can also be used in patients with more moderate hypercholesterolemia. Because their mechanism of action complements that of the statins and nicotinic acid, resins can be integral to many combination therapies, particularly for patients with severe primary hypercholesterolemia. Combining a fibrate with a statin is conceptually attractive for treating patients who require reduction in LDL-C and Tg levels, and an increase in HDL-C levels, but this combination has been associated with increased risk of diabetic myopathy and, rarely, rhabdomyolysis. In particular, the combination of gemfibrozil with a statin has been reported to increase the risk of diabetic myopathy and rhabdomyolysis. Combination therapy of ezetimibe/simvastatin (Vytorin®) is particularly effective in reducing LDL-C and minimizing statin dose, thus reducing the incidence of statin side effects.

## References

1.     Sprecher DL, Pearce GL: How deadly is the "deadly quartet"? *J Am Coll Cardiol* 2000;36:1159-1165.

2.     Gaede P, Vedel P, Larsen N, et al: Multifactorial intervention and cardiovascular disease in patients with type 2 diabetes. *N Engl J Med* 2003;348:383-393.

3.     Laakso M: Benefits of strict glucose and blood pressure control in type 2 diabetes: lessons from the UK Prospective Diabetes Study. *Circulation* 1999;99:461-462.

4.     Garber AJ: Treatment of hypertension in patients with diabetes mellitus. In: Taylor SI, ed: *Current Review of Diabetes*. Philadelphia, PA, Current Medicine Inc, 1999, pp 105-113.

5.     Fineberg SE: The treatment of hypertension and dyslipidemia in diabetes mellitus. *Prim Care* 1999;26:951-964.

6.     Arauz-Pacheco C, Parrott MA, Raskin P, and the American Diabetes Association: Treatment of hypertension in adults with diabetes. *Diabetes Care* 2003;26(suppl 1):S80-S82.

7.     Yusuf S, Sleight P, Pogue J, et al: Effects of an angiotensin-converting-enzyme inhibitor, ramipril, on cardiovascular events in high-risk patients. The Heart Outcomes Prevention Evaluation Study Investigators. *N Engl J Med* 2000;342:145-153.

8.     Fox KM, and European Trial on Reduction of Cardiac Events With Perindopril in Stable Coronary Artery Disease Investigators:

Efficacy of perindopril in reduction of cardiovascular events among patients with stable coronary artery disease: randomised, double-blind, placebo-controlled, multicentre trial (the EUROPA study). *Lancet* 2003;362:782-788.

9.    Lewis EJ, Hunsicker LG, Clarke WR, et al, and the Collaborative Study Group: Renoprotective effect of the angiotensin-receptor antagonist irbesartan in patients with nephropathy due to type 2 diabetes. *N Engl J Med* 2001;345:851-860.

10.    Brenner BM, Cooper ME, de Zeeuw D, et al, and the RENAAL Study Investigators: Effects of losartan on renal and cardiovascular outcomes in patients with type 2 diabetes and nephropathy. *N Engl J Med* 2001;345:861-869.

11.    Dahlof B, Devereux RB, Kjeldsen SE, et al, and the LIFE Study Group: Cardiovascular morbidity and mortality in the Losartan Intervention For Endpoint reduction in hypertension study (LIFE): a randomised trial against atenolol. *Lancet* 2002;359:995-1003.

12.    Cohn JN, Tognoni G, and the Balsartan Heart Failure Trial Investigators: A randomized trial of the angiotensin-receptor blocker valsartan in chronic heart failure. *N Engl J Med* 2001;345:1667-1675.

13.    Furberg CD, Psaty BM, Pahor M, et al: Clinical implications of recent findings from the Antihypertensive and Lipid-Lowering Treatment to Prevent Heart Attack Trial (ALLHAT) and other studies of hypertension. *Ann Intern Med* 2001;135:1074-1078.

14.    Cressman MD, Vidt DG, Mohler H, et al: Glucose tolerance during chronic propranolol treatment. *J Clin Hypertens* 1985;1:138-144.

15.    Bakris GL, Fonseca V, Katholi RE, et al, and the GEMINI Iinvestigators: Metabolic effects of carvedilol vs metoprolol in patients with type 2 diabetes mellitus and hypertension. *JAMA* 2004; 292:2227-2236.

16.    Grossman E, Messerli FH, Goldbourt U: High blood pressure and diabetes mellitus: are all antihypertensive drugs created equal? *Arch Intern Med* 2000;160:2447-2452.

17.    Furberg CD: Hypertension and diabetes: current issues. *Am Heart J* 1999;138:S400-S405.

18.    ALLHAT Officers and Coordinators for the ALLHAT Collaborative Research Group. The Antihypertensive and Lipid Lowering Treatment to Prevent Heart Attack Trial: Major outcomes in high-risk hypertensive patients randomized to angiotensin-converting enzyme inhibitor or calcium-channel blocker vs diuretic: The Antihyperten-

sive and Lipid-Lowering Treatment to Prevent Heart Attack Trial (ALLHAT). *JAMA* 2002;288:2981-2997.

19.  Neutel JM: The use of combination drug therapy in the treatment of hypertension. *Prog Cardiovasc Nurs* 2002;17:81-88.

20.  Hart PD, Bakris GL: Combination therapy for hypertension and renal disease in diabetes. In: Mogensen CE, ed: *The Kidney and Hypertension in Diabetes Mellitus*, 6th ed. London, England, Taylor & Francis, 2004.

21.  Fineberg SE: The treatment of hypertension and dyslipidemia in diabetes mellitus. *Prim Care* 1999;26:951-964.

22.  Expert Panel on Detection, Evaluation, and Treatment of High Blood Cholesterol in Adults: Executive Summary of the Third Report of the National Cholesterol Education Program (NCEP) Expert Panel on Detection, Evaluation, and Treatment of High Blood Cholesterol in Adults (Adult Treatment Panel III). *JAMA* 2001;285:2486-2497.

23.  Best JD, O'Neal DN: Diabetic dyslipidemia: current treatment recommendations. *Drugs* 2000;59:1101-1111.

24.  Illingworth DR: Management of hypercholesterolemia. *Med Clin North Am* 2000;84:23-42.

25.  Marcus AO: Lipid disorders in patients with type 2 diabetes. Meeting the challenges of early, aggressive treatment. *Postgrad Med* 2001;110:111-114, 117-118, 121-123.

26.  Frick MH, Elo O, Haapa K, et al: Helsinki Heart Study: primary-prevention trial with gemfibrozil in middle-aged men with dyslipidemia: safety of treatment, changes in risk factors, and incidence of coronary heart disease. *N Engl J Med* 1987;317:1237-1245.

27.  Rubins HB, Robins SJ, Collins D, et al. Gemfibrozil for the secondary prevention of coronary heart disease in men with low levels of high-density lipoprotein cholesterol: Veterans Affairs High-Density Lipoprotein Cholesterol Intervention Trial Study Group. *N Engl J Med* 1999;341:410-418.

28.  Keech A, Simes RJ, Barter P, et al, and The FIELD study investigators. Effects of long-term fenofibrate therapy on cardiovascular events in 9795 people with type 2 diabetes mellitus (the FIELD study): randomised controlled trial. *Lancet* 2005;366:1849-1861.

29.  Zetia® (ezetimibe) Annotated Prescribing Information. Merck/Schering-Plough Pharmaceuticals Inc, North Wales, PA, 2002.

# Chapter 10

# Microvascular Complications — Prevention and Management

## Diabetic Retinopathy

Diabetic retinopathy (DR) is the leading cause of blindness in adults younger than age 65, despite highly effective treatment strategies developed over the past several decades. Diabetic patients are 25 times more likely to develop blindness than the general population.[1] In the United States alone, DR results in blindness of >10,000 patients with diabetes per year.[2] Proliferative retinopathy and macular edema are the primary causes of blindness in diabetic patients, along with the increased incidence of cataracts and glaucoma.[3] According to the most recent estimate, approximately 5.5 million adult patients with diabetes have DR.[4] DR is more common in patients with type 1 diabetes than type 2 diabetes. During the first two decades of disease, nearly all patients with type 1 diabetes and >60% of patients with type 2 diabetes develop DR. Unlike type 1 diabetes, in which vision-threatening retinopathy is rare in the first 3 to 5 years of diabetes or before puberty, there is evidence that DR begins to develop in patients at least 7 years before the formal diagnosis of type 2 diabetes.[5]

### Natural History

DR can be classified into several types (Table 10-1) and has an orderly course of progression beginning with mild nonproliferative abnormalities, characterized by increased vascular permeability, to moderate and severe nonproliferative diabetic retinopathy (NPDR), characterized by vascular closure, to proliferative diabetic retinopathy (PDR), characterized by the growth of new blood vessels on the retina and the posterior surface of the vitreous.[6] Macular edema, characterized by retinal thickening from leaky blood vessels, can develop at all stages of DR.[7]

Vision loss due to DR results from several mechanisms. Central vision may be impaired by macular edema or capillary nonperfusion. New blood vessels of PDR and contraction of the accompanying fibrous tissue can distort the retina and lead to tractional retinal detachment, producing severe and often irreversible vision loss. In addition, the new fragile blood vessels tend to bleed and cause preretinal or vitreous hemorrhage. In diabetic patients with PDR, these vitreous hemorrhages are the leading cause of severe vision loss.

### Diagnosis and Screening Guidelines

A well-organized DR screening approach results in enormous benefits for patients and savings of millions of dollars in health-care costs (Table 10-2). For example, annual screening for DR in both type 1 diabetics without DR and follow-up every 6 months for those with DR, accompanied by appropriate treatment would result in a savings of 70,000 to 80,000 person-years of sight and $60 to $80 million annually in the United States.[8] In the case of type 2 diabetes, these numbers are >94,000 person-years of sight and >$250 million/year.[9]

Patients with type 1 diabetes should have an initial dilated and comprehensive eye examination by an ophthalmologist or optometrist within 3 to 5 years after the onset of diabetes. Because changes as the result of DR may be present many years before the diagnosis of type 2 diabetes, patients with type 2 diabetes should have an initial dilated

**Table 10-1: Classifications
of Diabetic Retinopathy**

**Classification**

Background (nonproliferative) retinopathy

Background retinopathy with maculopathy

Proliferative retinopathy

Advanced diabetic eye disease

Involutional retinopathy

and comprehensive eye examination by an ophthalmologist or optometrist shortly after diabetes diagnosis.

Subsequently, both type 1 and type 2 diabetes patients should have a comprehensive eye examination by an ophthalmologist or optometrist annually or more frequently once DR begins to progress. Patients with any level of macular edema, severe NPDR, or PDR require the prompt care of an ophthalmologist who is knowledgeable and experienced in the management and treatment of DR. Referral to an ophthalmologist should not be delayed until PDR has developed in patients who are known to have severe nonproliferative or more

| Characteristics | Impact on Vision |
| --- | --- |
| Microaneurysms, venous dilatation, hemorrhages, exudates | None |
| Macular edema | May impair vision |
| Neovascularization (pathognomonic feature), fibrous proliferation, preretinal hemorrhage, vitreous hemorrhage | Vision already affected at this stage |
| Vitreous opacities (hemorrhage and fibrous tissues), retinal detachment | Vision already affected at this stage |
| Residual scarring from previously active proliferative diabetic retinopathy (PDR) | Vision already affected at this stage |

advanced DR because laser treatment at this stage is associated with a 50% reduction in the risk of severe visual loss and vitrectomy.

### Pregnancy

DR frequently worsens during pregnancy for diabetic women. When planning a pregnancy, diabetic women should have a comprehensive eye examination and should be counseled on the risk of development and/or progression of DR. Women with diabetes who become pregnant should have a comprehensive eye examination in the first trimester and close follow-up throughout pregnancy.

## Table 10-2: Screening Guidelines for Diabetic Retinopathy

**Patient Group**

Type 1 diabetes

Type 2 diabetes

Pregnancy in patients with pre-existing diabetes

## Risk Factors for Development and Progression of Diabetic Retinopathy

### Duration of Diabetes

A well-established linear relation exists between duration of diabetes and the presence and severity of DR. For example, the Wisconsin Epidemiologic Study of Diabetic Retinopathy (WESDR)[10] found that 3.6% of patients with type 1 diabetes whose disease onset occurred before age 30 were legally blind, compared with 1.6% of patients with type 2 diabetes whose disease onset occurred after age 30.

### Poor Glycemic Control

The most effective treatment to slow the progression of DR is good glycemic control. Both the Diabetes Control and Complications Trial (DCCT) in type 1 diabetics[11] and the United Kingdom Prospective Diabetes Study (UKPDS) in type 2 diabetics[12] conclusively showed the efficacy of good glycemic control in preventing DR. In the DCCT, after a mean follow-up of 6.5 years, the group of patients treated with intensive insulin therapy and had a mean glycosylated hemoglobin $A_{1c}$ (Hb$A_{1c}$) of 7.2% showed reduced

| Recommended First Examination | Follow-up Examination |
|---|---|
| Within 3-5 years after diagnosis of diabetes once patient is age 10 years or older | Yearly |
| At time of diagnosis of diabetes | Yearly |
| Prior to conception and during first trimester | Physician discretion pending results of first-trimester examination |

progression of DR or delayed development of DR by 27% compared with patients treated with nonintensive therapy, but, in the UKPDS, intensive glycemic control therapy reduced microvascular complications including DR by 25% compared with conventional therapy. Furthermore, the UKPDS also showed a continuous relationship between the risk of microvascular complications and the degree of glycemic control. Every percentage point decrease in $HbA_{1c}$ was associated with 35% risk reduction.

The effort to achieve good glycemic control in diabetics should be a priority from the time of diagnosis because the benefit of glycemic control declines substantially in patients with advanced DR.[13]

**Elevated Blood Pressure**

Epidemiologic studies suggest that hypertension increases the risk of development and progression of DR and macular edema. In the WESDR, higher diastolic blood pressure was associated with increased progression of DR and macular edema. In the UKPDS, type 2 diabetics with blood pressure of <150/85 had a 34% reduction in progression of DR and a 47% reduced risk of deterioration in visual acuity compared with patients with blood pressure <185/105.[14]

Hypertension impairs the autoregulation of retinal blood flow in diabetics compared with nondiabetics. It also enhances the endothelial damage and expression of vascular endothelial growth factor (VEGF) and its receptors in poorly controlled diabetics.[15]

## Hyperlipidemia

Effects of serum lipids on DR and macular edema are still under investigation. The WESDR[17] showed an association between elevated serum lipids levels and more severe retinal hard exudates, a significant risk factor for moderate vision loss. Similarly, the Early Treatment Diabetic Retinopathy Study (ETDRS) showed an association between elevated baseline low-density lipoprotein (LDL) levels and retinal hard exudates.[16] In addition, retinal hard exudate development was 50% more likely in patients with elevated total cholesterol or triglycerides (Tgs).[17]

## Diabetic Nephropathy and Anemia

Type 1 diabetes patients with diabetic nephropathy almost always have DR; even patients who have microalbuminuria are at increased risk of DR.[18] Common predisposing factors, such as chronic hyperglycemia, duration of diabetes, and hypertension, most likely account for this relationship in type 1 diabetes.

The relationship between diabetic nephropathy and DR is not as strong in type 2 diabetes. In one study of type 2 diabetics with significant proteinuria, 77% had diabetic nephropathy while only 56% of those patients had DR.[19]

Renal failure often results in anemia; epidemiologically, anemia is the second greatest risk factor for the development and rapid progression of DR. The ETDRS found that low hematocrit was an independent risk factor for high-risk PDR and vision loss.

## Pregnancy

Diabetic women who begin a pregnancy without DR at conception carry a 10% risk of developing NPDR, whereas 4% of diabetic women with NPDR develop PDR during pregnancy. Women who begin pregnancy with poor glycemic control and then achieve control also develop PDR rapidly, which may not improve completely after pregnancy.[20]

## *Treatment of Diabetic Retinopathy*
### Medical Therapy

Medical therapy has a controversial place in the management of DR. To date neither aspirin[21] nor ticlopidine (Ticlid®)[22] has shown any definitive benefits.

### Surgical Treatment

The success of laser photocoagulation in the treatment of DR is well established. Two types of laser treatment are in use: focal (or direct), and panretinal (or scatter). Focal therapy, in which small areas of macular tissue with leakage are directly treated with moderately intense photoenergy, is used for the treatment of macular edema.[23]

Panretinal treatment, also known as grid therapy, is the treatment of choice for advanced DR. In this treatment, 1,500 to 2,000 laser burns are applied in a polka-dotted pattern.

The mechanism of action of panretinal treatment is unknown. Some investigators believe that it decreases the production of vasoproliferative factors by eliminating a portion of the hypoxic retina[24] or by stimulating the release of antiangiogenic factors from the retinal pigment epithelium.[25] The number of burns necessary to achieve this effect has not been established.

### Vitrectomy

Vitrectomy involves removal of the opaque vitreous humor followed by photocoagulation to the retina.[26]

Vitrectomy is generally recommended if laser treatment fails to inhibit new vessel proliferation. Other indications for vitrectomy include the presence of tractional macular detachment, combined tractional and rhematogenous (ruptured) retinal detachment, progressive fibrovascular proliferation, dense premacular hemorrhage, neovascularization of the iris (rubeosis iridis) with vitreous hemorrhage, and cataracts with PDR.[27]

### *Prevention of Diabetic Retinopathy*

Strong clinical data from the DCCT, Epidemiology of Diabetes Interventions and Complications (EDIC) study, and the UKPDS studies suggest that DR can be prevented by strict glycemic control. In addition, control of blood pressure and hyperlipidemia, and early detection and aggressive management of microalbuminuria and anemia, can slow the onset and progression of DR.

## Diabetic Nephropathy

Diabetic nephropathy is a clinical syndrome characterized by persistent albuminuria of >300 mg/24 hours, high blood pressure, and progressive decline in glomerular filtration rate (GFR) in the absence of other known renal diseases. Diabetic nephropathy, although uncommon in type 1 diabetics in the first 5 years after diagnosis, affects up to 35% of patients with type 1 diabetes and 20% of type 2 diabetics.[28] All patients with type 1 diabetes with nephropathy also have DR, whereas DR is present in only 50% to 70% of type 2 diabetics at the time of diagnosis of nephropathy.

Diabetic nephropathy is the leading cause of end-stage renal disease (ESRD) in the United States, accounting for 28,000 new cases/year. Patients with diabetic nephropathy who are on dialysis have a 22% higher mortality rate at 1 year and 15% at 5 years than patients without diabetes.[28] In 2005, the cost of care for a diabetic patient undergoing dialysis was $74,177/year, which was approximately

$12,500 more than patients without diabetes. Diabetic nephropathy confers a high risk of not only ESRD, but also cardiovascular morbidity and mortality.[28]

## Risk Factors for the Development and Progression of Diabetic Nephropathy

There are multiple risk factors for the development and progression of diabetic nephropathy in both type 1 and type 2 diabetics.

1. **Genetic predisposition:** For both type 1 and type 2 diabetics, a family history of diabetic nephropathy in a sibling or parent increases the likelihood of developing nephropathy.[29]

2. **Ethnicity:** Blacks have three to six times increased incidence of diabetic nephropathy compared with nonblacks. Nephropathy is also more severe among blacks.[30]

3. **Age:** Epidemiologic evidence suggests that older age at the time of diagnosis of type 2 diabetes is associated with increased risk for developing diabetic nephropathy.[31]

4. **Duration of diabetes:** The onset of overt nephropathy in type 1 diabetes is typically between 10 and 15 years after the onset of the disease. Those patients who have no proteinuria after 20 to 25 years only have about a 1% risk/year of developing overt renal disease.[32] In the case of type 2 diabetes, this association is less well established due to delayed diagnosis, although there are ample data to suggest that the time to proteinuria from the onset of diabetes and the time to ESRD from the onset of proteinuria are similar in both type 1 and type 2 diabetes.[33]

5. **Obesity:** A high body mass index (BMI) is associated with an increased risk of chronic kidney disease (CKD) among patients with diabetes.[31]

6. **Glycemic control:** A close correlation between mean $HbA_{1c}$ level and overt nephropathy is well established. Diabetic nephropathy is more likely to develop in patients with worse glycemic control (higher $HbA_{1c}$ levels).[33]

10

7. **Blood-pressure control:** Thirty percent of type 2 diabetics have high blood pressure at the time of diagnosis, and this number increases to 70% with onset of nephropathy.[34] High blood pressure accelerates the development of microalbuminuria and loss of renal function in previously stable patients.

8. **Lipid control:** Twenty percent of patients with type 2 diabetes have ischemic nephropathy secondary to atherosclerosis of the abdominal aorta with renal artery stenosis or cholesterol microembolism, and diabetic patients with elevated cholesterol or Tgs have a faster decline in renal function than patients without such elevations.[34]

9. **Smoking:** The ability of smoking to accelerate diabetic nephropathy is well established. Although smoking cessation has not been proven to have a renoprotective effect in type 2 diabetics, it clearly reduces cardiovascular risk and slows the loss of renal function in type 1 diabetics.[34]

### *Natural History and Pathophysiology of Diabetic Nephropathy*

Diabetic nephropathy runs a smoldering course, and initial stages are completely asymptomatic. Microalbuminuria is the first biochemical evidence of its onset. Diabetic nephropathy can be arbitrarily divided into the following stages:

1. **Glomerular hyperfiltration:** Despite good glycemic control, 25% to 40% of diabetic patients show glomerular hyperfiltration with a higher rate of progression to clinical diabetic nephropathy compared with diabetics without hyperfiltration. This hemodynamic change appears to be due to dilatation of the afferent (precapillary) glomerular arteriole, which plays an important role in the hyperfiltration response, by raising both the intraglomerular pressure and renal blood flow.[35]

2. **Early glomerular lesions:** Mild thickening of the glomerular basement membrane appears after 3 to 5

years of onset of diabetes and is assumed to be secondary to glycosylation of basement membrane proteins. Exercise-induced microalbuminuria is the only clinical evidence of renal involvement at this stage.[36]

3. **Microalbuminuria:** Microalbuminuria is defined by a daily urinary excretion rate of 20 to 200 µg/min and heralds the clinical onset of renal deterioration and vascular damage in other organs.

4. **Clinical diabetic nephropathy:** Progression to macroalbuminuria and falling GFR sets in after 15 to 20 years of diabetes onset. Nephrotic syndrome is also common at this stage.[37]

5. **End-stage renal disease:** Without intervention, uremic symptoms with rising creatinine level are the hallmark of this stage and patients will need dialysis within the next 2 to 3 years.[38]

### Diagnosis of Diabetic Nephropathy

Given the high morbidity and mortality associated with diabetic nephropathy, guidelines for screening have been established for early detection and intervention to prevent the condition or slow its progression.

The American Diabetes Association (ADA) recommends a yearly screening for individuals with type 2 diabetes and a yearly screening for those with type 1 diabetes after 5 years' duration of disease.[39] Several screening techniques are available. Use of the urine albumin-to-creatinine ratio in an untimed urinary sample is recommended as the preferred screening strategy for all diabetic patients,[39] but a 24-hour urine collection for albuminuria and creatinine, or a timed (eg, overnight or 3- to 4-hour) urine collection are also acceptable. Positive results need to be confirmed with a second measurement because of the high variability in urinary albumin excretion in people with diabetes. Microalbuminuria is considered to be present if urinary albumin excretion is 30 to 300 mg/24 hours (equivalent to 20 to 200 µg/min on a timed specimen or 30 to 300 mg/g

## Table 10-3: Interpretation of Urinary Albumin Excretion Findings*

| Finding | Urinary AER (μg/min) | Urinary AER (mg/24 hr) |
|---|---|---|
| Normal | <20 | <30 |
| Microalbuminuria | 20-200 | 30-300 |
| Macroalbuminuria | >200 | >300 |

*Based on different assessment methods.

AER=albumin excretion rate in a timed specimen

From Standards of Medical Care in Diabetes Recommendations 2007: *Diabetes Care* 2007;30(suppl 1):S4-S41.[39]

creatinine on a random sample) (Table 10-3). Short-term hyperglycemia, exercise, urinary tract infections (UTIs), marked hypertension, heart failure, and acute febrile illness can cause transient elevations in urinary albumin excretion.[40] There is also marked day-to-day variability in urinary albumin excretion, so at least two to three collections done in a 3- to 6-month period should show elevated albumin levels before a patient is designated as having microalbuminuria and treatment is initiated.

### *Prevention and Treatment Strategies for Diabetic Nephropathy*
### General Measures

The early detection of diabetic nephropathy and timely pharmacologic intervention can result in the regression of nephropathy.[41,42] Lifestyle modifications, including weight loss, exercise, smoking cessation, and reduced alcohol and sodium intake should receive special emphasis in patients at high risk of developing diabetic nephropathy. Diabetic

| Urine-albumin-to-creatinine ratio (mg/g) | Morning urine albumin concentration (mg/L) |
|:---:|:---:|
| <30 | <30 |
| 30-300 | 30-300 |
| >300 | >300 |

patients should obtain 10% to 20% of their daily caloric intake from protein, as studies have shown that protein consumption in the range of 0.5 to 0.85 g/kg/day significantly reduces the rate of decline in GFR or creatinine clearance ($C_{cr}$) in type 1 diabetics, although equally compelling data for patients with type 2 diabetes are not available.[43]

**Renoprotective Pharmacotherapies**

In addition to optimal glycemic control, achieving blood-pressure control can have a major impact on the evolution and progression of diabetic nephropathy. Use of angiotensin-converting enzyme (ACE) inhibitors, or, more recently, angiotensin receptor blockers (ARBs) has become the standard of care in patients with diabetes.[44]

**Use of ACE inhibitors:** The value of ACE inhibitors in patients with established diabetic nephropathy was demonstrated in the landmark Diabetic Retinopathy Study (DRS) with captopril (Capoten®).[45] Four hundred and nine patients with overt proteinuria and creatinine ≤2.5 mg/dL were randomized to therapy with either captopril or placebo. With equivalent blood-pressure control, patients treated with captopril had a slower rate of increase in creatinine concentration and a lesser likelihood of progression to ESRD or death.[45] Captopril treatment was also associated with a 50% reduction in the risk of the combined end points of death, dialysis, and kidney transplantation that was independent of blood pressure.

The data are fragmented on the effect of antihypertensive therapy with ACE inhibitors in patients with diabetic nephropathy caused by type 2 diabetes, although a similar benefit seems to be present. More data from large clinical trials are available on the efficacy of ARBs. In the UKPDS, each 10 mm Hg reduction in systolic blood pressure was associated with a 12% risk reduction in diabetic complications ($P$ <0.001); the lowest risk occurred at a systolic blood pressure <120 mm Hg. There was no difference between captopril and atenolol (Tenormin®) in progression of complications.[46] Similar results were found in the Antihypertensive and Lipid-Lowering Treatment to Prevent Heart Attack Trial (ALLHAT)[47]; however, the Heart Outcomes Prevention Evaluation (HOPE) trial showed decreased proteinuria with ACE inhibitors.[48]

**Use of angiotensin blockers:** In the Irbesartan Diabetic Nephropathy Trial (IDNT), the angiotensin II receptor blocker irbesartan (Avapro®) was effective in protecting against the progression of diabetic nephropathy caused by type 2 diabetes. This protection was independent of the reduction in blood pressure observed with irbesartan.[49] Irbesartan was also shown to be renoprotective independently of its blood-pressure-lowering effect in patients with type 2 diabetes and microalbuminuria, slowing the progression to overt proteinuria.[49]

In the Reduction in End Points in Noninsulin-Dependent Diabetes Mellitus with the Angiotensin II Antagonist Losartan (RENAAL) trial,[50] losartan (Cozaar®) significantly reduced the incidence of a doubling of the serum creatinine concentration (risk reduction=25%) and ESRD (risk reduction=28%), but had no effect on the mortality rate. The benefit exceeded that attributable to changes in blood pressure. The composite of morbidity and mortality from cardiovascular causes was similar in both groups, although the rate of first hospitalization for heart failure was significantly lower with losartan (risk reduction=32%). The level of proteinuria declined by 35% with losartan.[50]

**Combination of ACE inhibitors and ARBs:** Many short-term studies demonstrate a greater reduction in protein excretion in diabetic nephropathy with combination ACE inhibitors and ARBs compared with monotherapy with an ACE inhibitor or an ARB alone. One randomized trial of 199 patients with type 2 diabetes and hypertension (baseline blood pressure=160/95 mm Hg) and microalbuminuria (but normal kidney function) demonstrated a greater reduction in albuminuria with combination therapy (candesartan [Atacand®] and lisinopril [Prinivil®, Zestril®]) compared with either agent alone.[51] Patients were initially assigned to either agent alone, and after 12 weeks, half of the patients in each group had the other agent added. After an additional 12 weeks, patients in the combination candesartan and lisinopril groups had 50%, 24%, and 39% reductions in albuminuria, respectively, and 15/16, 14/10, and 17/10 mm Hg reductions in blood pressure, respectively.

*Aldosterone antagonists:* Spironolactone (Aldactone®) appears to reduce proteinuria when used alone and to have an additive effect on proteinuria when used in combination with an ACE inhibitor or an ARB in both type 1 and type 2 diabetes. Lowering of blood pressure and anti-inflammatory actions are the proposed mechanisms for these beneficial effects.[52] There are no long-term data regarding benefit with the combination of ACE inhibitor or ARB and aldosterone blockade in terms of slowing the rate of loss of GFR. The risk of inducing or aggravating hyperkalemia in patients with long-standing diabetic nephropathy may limit the use of aldosterone antagonists.

*β-**Blockers and Calcium-Channel Blockers:*** β-Blockers have shown a variable response in the treatment of diabetic nephropathy. β-Blockers decrease the protein excretion rate, although to a substantially lesser degree than ACE inhibitors or ARBs.[53]

Among the calcium-channel blockers (CCBs), only the use of diltiazem (Cardizem®, Dilacor XR®) and verapamil (Calan®, Covera-HS®, Isoptin® SR, Verelan®) have consistently been shown to decrease urinary protein excretion in patients with diabetic nephropathy. In addition, their use in combination with ACE inhibitors has demonstrated an additive effect.[54]

## Treatment of Advanced Diabetic Nephropathy

Once macroalbuminuria develops, ESRD is almost inevitable. Once GFR declines to <60, serum creatinine is elevated, indicating low clearance. A nephrology referral is mandatory at this point because this stage of diabetic nephropathy is difficult to manage due to the presence of other complications including cardiovascular disease (CVD) and osteodystrophy. In addition, the pharmacokinetics of insulin and other medications change for these patients because of decreased renal metabolism and clearance. Metformin (Glucophage®, Glucophage® XR, Glumetza™) is contraindicated, and thiazolidinediones (TZDs) become difficult to use because of fluid retention. Both hypoglycemia and hyperglycemia frequently occur.

## Renal Replacement Therapy

A serum creatinine level of ≥4 mg/dL warrants consideration and planning of renal replacement therapy. Diabetic patients are candidates for all three types of renal replacement therapy: hemodialysis, peritoneal dialysis, and kidney transplantation. In general, patients have equal outcomes with peritoneal and hemodialysis but better outcomes with transplantation than dialysis.[55] For patients with type 1 diabetes, a combined kidney-pancreas transplantation produces better outcomes than kidney transplantation alone.[56]

## Diabetic Neuropathy

Diabetic neuropathy is defined as the presence of symptoms and/or signs of peripheral nerve dysfunction in people with diabetes after the exclusion of other causes. A careful history and physical examination are necessary to diagnose diabetic neuropathy, but absence of symptoms does not exclude the presence of neuropathy because asymptomatic neuropathy is common.[57] Diabetic neuropathies are the most common long-term complications of diabetes, affecting up to 50% of patients.[12] The duration of diabetes is the most important factor in frequency of neuropathy in patients with type 1 diabetes; however, diabetic neuropathy may be present at diagnosis of type 2 diabetes. There is evidence that the presence of diabetic neuropathy also portends an increased risk of mortality in diabetic patients. The presence of DR, poor glycemic control, and older age are other risk factors for the development of diabetic polyneuropathy.[58]

### Pathogenesis

The duration and severity of hyperglycemia is the most important factor in the development and progression of diabetic neuropathy. Improving hyperglycemia by intensive insulin therapy or pancreatic transplantation improves diabetic neuropathy in patients with type 1 diabetes. However, in type 2 diabetes, the role of intensive insulin treatment and its effect on the improvement in neuropathy is controversial. Other proposed factors involved in the pathogenesis of diabetic neuropathy include the polyol pathway, myoinositol deficiency, oxidative stress, advanced glycation end products (AGEs), and immune mechanisms.[58]

### *Classification of Diabetic Neuropathy*

This chapter uses the classification based on the premise that diabetic neuropathy is not a single condition but the

## Table 10-4: Classification of Diabetic Neuropathy

*Rapidly reversible hyperglycemic neuropathy*
*Generalized symmetric diabetic polyneuropathy*

- Sensorimotor (chronic)
- Acute sensory
- Autonomic

*Focal and multifocal neuropathies*

- Cranial
- Thoracolumbar radiculoneuropathy
- Focal limb
- Proximal motor (amyotrophy)
- Superimposed chronic inflammatory demyelinating neuropathy

result of a number of disturbances in the peripheral nervous system as a consequence of hyperglycemia (Table 10-4).[59]

**Rapidly Reversible Hyperglycemic Neuropathy**

Rapidly reversible abnormalities of nerve conduction may occur in patients with recently diagnosed or transient poorly controlled diabetes; these abnormalities may be accompanied by distal uncomfortable sensory symptoms. Such changes are unlikely to be caused by structural abnormalities because recovery soon follows restoration of euglycemia. It remains unknown whether these temporary abnormalities result in a greater risk of developing other chronic neuropathies in later life.[60]

**Generalized Symmetric Diabetic Polyneuropathy**

Acute sensory neuropathy is a distinct variety of the symmetric polyneuropathies with an acute or subacute onset characterized by severe sensory symptoms, usually with few, if any, clinical signs. The natural history is one of gradual improvement of these symptoms with positive changes in glycemic control.

Pain is the most common complaint in all patients, who may also experience severe weight loss, depression, and, frequently in men, erectile dysfunction (ED). Other commonly reported symptoms include constant burning discomfort (especially in the feet), severe hyperesthesias, and deep aching pain, and many experience sudden, sharp, stabbing, or electric shock-like sensations in the lower limbs. All symptoms are prone to nocturnal exacerbation, with bed clothes irritating hyperesthetic skin.

Rarely, diabetic neuropathy may develop after sudden improvement of glycemic control; the term insulin neuritis is a misnomer because it can also follow improvement of glycemic control induced by oral hypoglycemic agents. These observations are in keeping with the hypothesis that plasma-glucose flux is important in the genesis of neuropathic pain.[59]

Chronic sensorimotor neuropathy, a subtype of diabetic peripheral neuropathy (DPN), is the most common form of diabetic neuropathy. It is usually of insidious onset and may be present at the diagnosis of type 2 diabetes in >10% of subjects. As in acute sensory neuropathy, painful symptoms tend to be more pronounced at night, but in addition, patients with this form of neuropathy may experience negative symptoms, such as numbness. Patients often mention unsteady gait due to disturbed proprioception and possibly abnormal muscle sensory function.[61] Such unsteadiness has been quantified and may result in repetitive minor trauma or falls, and in late complications, such as trauma or Charcot's neuroarthropathy.

Upon clinical examination, there is usually a symmetric sensory loss to all modalities in a stocking distribution. In severe cases, this may extend well above the ankle and involve the hands. The ankle reflexes are usually reduced

10

## Table 10-5: Classification of Diabetic Autonomic Neuropathy

*Cardiovascular*

- Reduced heart rate variability
- Exercise intolerance
- Orthostatic hypotension
- Silent (or painless) myocardial ischemia

*Gastrointestinal*

- Esophageal dysfunction
- Gastroparesis
- Constipation
- Diarrhea
- Fecal incontinence

*Genitourinary*

- Cystopathy
- Neurogenic bladder
- Erectile dysfunction (ED)
- Female sexual dysfunction

*Skin*

- Hyperhidrosis
- Anhidrosis

*Metabolic*

- Hypoglycemic unawareness and unresponsiveness

or absent, and the knee reflexes may also be absent in some cases. Motor weakness is unusual, although small muscle wasting in the feet and also in the hands may be seen in more advanced cases. Any pronounced motor signs should raise the possibility of a nondiabetic etiology of the neuropathy, especially if the neuropathy is asymmetric. Romberg's sign may be present in severe cases. Chronic sensorimotor neuropathy is often accompanied by autonomic neuropathy.

### Diabetic Autonomic Neuropathy

Diabetic autonomic neuropathy (DAN) can cause dysfunction of any system of the body and can occur as early as 1 year after the diagnosis of type 2 diabetes. Despite its negative impact on survival and quality of life (QOL), DAN often goes unrecognized for a long time because of its insidious onset and complex, vague multiorgan symptoms. The most common and well-recognized symptoms and signs of DAN are listed in Table 10-5.

### Cardiac Autonomic Neuropathy

Cardiac autonomic neuropathy (CAN) results from damage to the autonomic nerve fibers that innervate the heart and blood vessels, and results in abnormalities in heart rate control and vascular dynamics. Patients with CAN have a five times higher mortality rate compared with diabetics without CAN.[62]

**Reduced heart rate variability and exercise intolerance:** Reduced heart rate variation is the earliest indicator of CAN.[62] Lack of heart rate variability during deep breathing or exercise confers a high risk of coronary heart disease (CHD), regardless of the presence of diabetes. In patients with CAN, exercise intolerance results in reduced response in heart rate and blood pressure during exercise and decreased cardiac output predisposing these patients to cardiac ischemia. The severity of CAN correlates inversely with an increase in heart rate at any time during exercise and with the maximal increase in heart rate.[63]

**Orthostatic hypotension:** Orthostatic hypotension is defined as a decrease in blood pressure (ie, >20 mm Hg for systolic blood pressure or >10 mm Hg for diastolic blood

10

pressure) in response to postural change from supine to standing. In patients with diabetes, orthostatic hypotension is usually due to damage to the efferent sympathetic vasomotor fibers, particularly in the splanchnic vasculature. Patients with orthostatic hypotension typically present with lightheadedness and presyncopal symptoms. Symptoms, such as dizziness, weakness, fatigue, visual blurring, and neck pain, also may be due to orthostatic hypotension.[64]

**Silent (or painless) myocardial ischemia:** CAN may cause a decreased appreciation of chest pain and may also result in a delay in initiating appropriate therapy. Painless ischemia, which confers a greater risk of mortality after myocardial infarction (MI), occurs in 38% of patients with autonomic neuropathy, compared with 5% of those without such neuropathy.[65]

## Gastrointestinal Autonomic Neuropathy

Gastrointestinal (GI) disturbances (eg, esophageal enteropathy, gastroparesis, constipation, diarrhea, fecal incontinence) are common, and any section of the GI tract may be affected.

Esophageal dysfunction results at least in part from vagal neuropathy; symptoms include heartburn and dysphagia for solids. With the use of radioisotopic techniques that quantify gastric emptying, it appears that 50% of patients with longstanding diabetes have delayed gastric emptying (ie, gastroparesis).[66] Gastroparesis is a syndrome characterized by delayed gastric emptying in the absence of mechanical obstruction of the stomach. The cardinal symptoms include postprandial fullness (early satiety), nausea, vomiting, and bloating. Episodes of nausea or vomiting may last days to months or occur in cycles. Gastroparesis is one of the most debilitating of all diabetic GI complications because it usually results in nutritional compromise, impaired glucose control, and poor QOL, independently of other factors such as age, smoking, alcohol use, or type of diabetes.

Intermittent diarrhea is another discomforting outcome of DAN evident in 20% of diabetic patients. Bowel movements may occur ≥20 times/day with urgency, and the stools are often watery. Fecal incontinence due to poor sphincter tone is common for individuals with diabetes and may be associated with severe paroxysmal diarrhea or constitute an independent disorder of anorectal dysfunction.[67]

**Genitourinary Autonomic Neuropathy**

Neurogenic bladder, also called diabetic cystopathy, is a frequent complication of diabetes; as many as 45% of patients with diabetes exhibit diabetic cystopathy.[68] The prevalence rate of diabetic cystopathy increases with the duration of diabetes (25% in patients with diabetes of 10 years' duration, and >50% in patients with diabetes of 45 years' duration).[69]

Diabetic cystopathy is characterized by impaired sensation of bladder fullness, increased bladder capacity, reduced bladder contractility, and increased postvoid residual urine (PVR).

Diabetic cystopathy causes secondary complications such as UTIs, vesicoureteral reflux, and hydroureteronephrosis caused by prolonged urinary retention. Pyelonephritis, nephrolithiasis, and sometimes urosepsis can develop. Finally, uremia may develop after continuing damage to kidney function due to diabetic glomerulosclerosis. Urinary frequency is another commonly associated symptom of autonomic dysfunction of the genitourinary system. Unfortunately, 37% to 50% of individuals with diabetes have symptoms of bladder dysfunction, and 43% to 87% of individuals with type 1 diabetes have physiologic evidence of bladder dysfunction.[70]

**Sexual Dysfunction**

ED is the most common form of organic sexual dysfunction in men with diabetes, with an incidence estimated to be between 35% and 75%.[71] Etiology of ED in diabetes is multifactorial, including neuropathy, vascular disease, metabolic control, nutrition, endocrine disorders, psychogenic factors, and antidiabetes drugs. Retrograde ejaculation into the bladder also occurs in diabetic males.[72]

Women with diabetes may have decreased sexual desire and increased pain during intercourse and are at risk of decreased sexual arousal and inadequate lubrication.[73]

## Sweating Disturbances

Hyperhidrosis of the upper body, often related to eating (gustatory sweating), and anhidrosis of the lower body are characteristic features of autonomic neuropathy.[74] Gustatory sweating accompanies the ingestion of certain foods, particularly spicy foods and cheeses. Symptomatic relief can be obtained by avoiding the specific inciting food. Loss of lower body sweating can cause dry, brittle skin that cracks easily, predisposing one to ulcer formation that can lead to loss of a limb.

## Metabolic Concerns: Hypoglycemic Unawareness and Unresponsiveness

The absence of warning signs of impending neuroglycopenia is known as hypoglycemic unawareness. The failure of glucose counterregulation can be confirmed by the absence of glucagon and epinephrine responses to hypoglycemia induced by a standard, controlled dose of insulin. In patients with type 1 diabetes, the glucagon response is impaired with diabetes duration of 1 to 5 years, and, after 14 to 31 years of diabetes, the glucagon response is almost undetectable. It is not present in those with DAN. However, a syndrome of hypoglycemic autonomic failure occurs with the intensification of diabetes control and repeated episodes of hypoglycemia. The exact mechanism is not understood, but it does represent a real barrier to physiologic glycemic control.[75]

### *Focal and Multifocal Diabetic Neuropathies*

About 10% of diabetic neuropathies are focal or multifocal. Although the pain they cause may be severe, they have a good prognosis. Subtypes include cranial thoracolumbar, focal, and proximal motor (amytrophy), which have a combined prevalence of 3% to 36% in patients with diabetes.[76]

Focal limb diabetic neuropathies are often, but not always, due to entrapment (eg, carpal tunnel syndrome), indicating the greater susceptibility of diabetic nerve to compression. Among the cranial nerves, those supplying the external ocular muscles are most commonly involved. Thoracolumbar radiculoneuropathies may present with girdle-like pain, occasionally with motor weakness of abdominal wall muscles. Proximal motor neuropathy (amyotrophy) may be unilateral or asymmetrically bilateral with pain, wasting, and weakness that may be relatively acute at onset.

**Cranial Diabetic Neuropathies**

Cranial neuropathies in diabetic patients are extremely rare and occur in older individuals with a long duration of diabetes.

Ocular neuropathies affect cranial nerves III, IV, and VI.[77] The classic presentation of oculomotor nerve palsy is that of an acute-onset diplopia with ptosis, ipsilateral headache, and pupillary sparing. Resolution occurs over 2 to 5 months in the majority of patients with potential of recurrence. Management is expectant with strong reassurance to the patient for recovery. Maintaining optimal glycemic control as well as minimizing the other stronger risk factors for ischemia, including hypertension and hyperlipidemia, may aid recovery.

Facial neuropathy (Bell's palsy) causes acute-onset unilateral weakness of facial muscles, widening of the palpebral fissure, and secondary corneal irritation. This is accompanied by varying degrees of disturbance in taste and hyperacusis. The presence of hypertension and severity of paralysis at onset, but not diabetes, determines the degree of recovery at 1 year.[78] If the presentation is acute for <1 week, 7 to 14 days of prednisone may be administered.

Other cranial nerves that may be affected in diabetes are olfactory, optic, and trigeminal, although their involvement should always raise suspicion of nondiabetic etiology in diabetic patients. Hearing loss as a result of VIII nerve involvement has also been described.[79]

**Entrapment and Compression Diabetic Neuropathies**

Carpal tunnel syndrome is the most common entrapment neuropathy encountered in diabetic patients and occurs as a result of median nerve compression under the transverse carpal ligament. Painful paresthesias of the fingers may progress to a deep-seated ache, which radiates up the forearm or, rarely, the arm. Motor weakness is uncommon, but thenar muscle wasting occurs particularly in the elderly. Two common clinical tests include the Phalen test (forearms held vertically and hands held in complete flexion for 1 minute; the results are positive if paresthesias develop in the median territory within 30 to 60 seconds) or the Tinel test (percussion at the wrist and palm induces paresthesias in the median nerve territory), but they have a high false-positive rate.[80] Treatment options include wrist splints, injections of cortisone into the carpal tunnel, and surgical sectioning of the transverse carpal ligament, which provide variable degrees of pain relief but do not particularly benefit muscle wasting or sensory loss.

Ulnar neuropathy is the second most common entrapment neuropathy (2.1%) and occurs as a result of ulnar nerve compression immediately distal to the ulnar groove beneath the edge of the flexor carpi ulnaris aponeurosis in the cubital tunnel. Typical symptoms include painful paresthesias in the fourth and fifth digits associated with hypothenar and interosseous muscle wasting. Management of patients is primarily conservative, with patients advised to avoid pressure to this area because the results of surgery are poor.

Other mononeuropathies include radial neuropathy, common peroneal nerve, lateral cutaneous nerve of thigh (meralgia paraesthetica), sciatic nerve, and obutrator nerve.[76]

Diabetic amyotrophy (proximal motor neuropathy) typically occurs in patients with type 2 diabetes aged 50 to 60 years and presents with severe pain and unilateral or bilateral muscle weakness and atrophy in the proximal thigh muscles. The pathogenesis of diabetic amyotrophy is controversial. Management consists of pain control with anti-inflammatory agents, opioids, or tricyclic antidepressants (TCAs); resistant cases may respond to immunosuppressive therapy.[81]

Diabetic truncal radiculoneuropathy primarily affects middle-aged to elderly diabetic men. Pain is a primary feature and is acute in onset but may evolve over several months. It is aching or burning in quality, may be superimposed with lancinating stabs, and demonstrates nocturnal exacerbation with cutaneous hyperesthesia. It occurs in a girdle-like distribution over the lower thoracic or abdominal wall, usually with unilateral distribution but sometimes with bilateral distribution. On rare occasions, it may result in motor weakness with bulging of the abdominal wall. Profound weight loss may accompany the onset of symptoms. Clinical examination demonstrates heterogeneous neurologic findings ranging from no abnormality to sensory loss and hyperesthesia in a complete dermatomal pattern but sometimes only involves the distribution of the ventral or dorsal rami. Spontaneous resolution of symptoms generally occurs within 4 to 6 months.[60]

Chronic inflammatory demyelinating neuropathy (CIDP) is a severe and progressive, but treatable, polyneuropathy occasionally seen in diabetic patients. Nerve biopsies in CIDP demonstrate segmental demyelination

## Table 10-6: Investigations of Peripheral Diabetic Neuropathy

*Urine*
- Glucose, protein

*Hematology*
- Complete blood count (CBC)
- Erythrocyte sedimentation rate
- Vitamin $B_{12}$
- Folate

*Biochemistry*
- Fasting plasma glucose (FPG)
- Glycosylated hemoglobin $A_{1c}$ ($HbA_{1c}$) levels
- Renal functions
- Liver functions
- Thyroid-stimulating hormone (TSH)

*Neurophysiologic tests*
- Assessment of distal and proximal nerve stimulation

*Biochemistry*
- Serum protein electrophoresis
- Serum angiotensin enzyme

*Immunology*
- Antinuclear factor
- Antiextractable nuclear antigen antibodies (anti-Ro, anti-La)
- Antineutrophil cytoplasmic antigen antibodies

*Others*
- Nerve biopsy

and remyelination, onion bulbs, and inflammatory in-filtrates. There are increased numbers of macrophages, indicating that a macrophage-associated demyelination is a characteristic feature of CIDP. Treatment includes long-term immunomodulatory therapy with combinations of corticosteroids, azathioprine (Azasan®, Imuran®), plasmapheresis, and intravenous immunoglobulin (IVIG), resulting in rapid and substantial improvement in neurologic deficits.[82]

### Diagnostic Assessment and Testing

The diagnosis of diabetic neuropathy requires a thorough history and physical examination based on information and recommendations for screening and testing (Table 10-6).

Sensory evaluation should focus on symptoms that concern patients the most, such as pricking, tingling, sensation of electric shock, burning, aching, and throbbing. In addition to pain assessment, light touch, vibration, and position sense should be evaluated. Touch sensitivity is commonly measured by using monofilament testing. Although testing with a 10-g monofilament can predict foot ulceration, as can Achilles reflex assessment, use of a 1-g monofilament increases sensitivity in detecting early neuropathy from 60% to 90%. Vibration perception should be measured with a 128-Hz tuning fork. Motor examination should evaluate muscular strength and reflexes.

### Treatment of Established Diabetic Neuropathies
#### Risk Factor Management

The pathogenesis of diabetic neuropathy involves multiple metabolic and vascular abnormalities that must be addressed simultaneously. A comprehensive approach including behavioral modification (ie, smoking cessation, moderate alcohol consumption), balanced nutrition, regular exercise, and pharmacologic therapy for hyperglycemia, hypertension, and hyperlipidemia can prevent or delay onset or worsening of diabetic neuropathy.

## Symptom Management by Neuropathy Type

**Pain management:** At any given time, up to 10% of diabetic patients with peripheral diabetic neuropathy have some form of pain that can be debilitating, but treatable. Duloxetine (Cymbalta®) and pregabalin (Lyrica®) are the only drugs approved by the US Food and Drug Administration (FDA) for the treatment of painful diabetic neuropathy.[83] In clinical practice, multiple medications (eg, nonsteroidal anti-inflammatory drugs [NSAIDs], muscle relaxants) are given a trial before prescribing duloxetine or pregabalin. The ADA recommends a sequential approach to the management of symptomatic diabetic polyneuropathy, which includes excluding nondiabetic causes, good glycemic control, use of antidepressant agents, use of anticonvulsant agents, use of $\alpha$-lipoic acid, use of opioid or opioid-like agents, and referral to a pain clinic. The ADA statement also approves use of nonpharmacologic, topical (acupuncture, capsaicin, glyceryl trinitrate spray or patches), or physical therapies.

Effective treatment of diabetic neuropathy remains inadequate. Improved glycemic control will improve nerve conduction velocity, but the symptoms of diabetic neuropathy may not necessarily improve. Avoidance of neurotoxins (eg, alcohol), supplementation with multivitamins for possible deficiencies, and symptomatic treatment are the mainstays of therapy. Foot ulceration, sepsis, and amputation are known and feared by almost every person who has diabetes. Foot complications develop in 25% of patients during their lifetime; consequently, prevention of such problems is of paramount importance. All diabetics should see a podiatrist at the time of their diagnosis and once a year thereafter. The pain of acute diabetic neuropathy may respond to over-the-counter analgesics, whereas chronic, painful diabetic neuropathy is difficult to treat but may respond to duloxetine, pregbalin, gabapentin (Neurontin®), TCAs, anticonvulsants (phenytoin [Dilantin®, Phenytek®], carbamazepine

[Carbatrol®, Equetro™, Tegretol®]), and capsaicin cream. Aldose reductase inhibitors and ACE inhibitors also may provide some relief. Referral to a pain management center may be necessary.

**Transcutaneous electrical nerve stimulation:** In patients who continue to have pain despite combination drug therapy, use of transcutaneous electrical nerve stimulation (TENS) units or a series of local nerve blocks have demonstrated some pain relief.[83]

**Surgical decompression:** Surgical decompression of multiple peripheral nerves (ie, the Dellon procedure) is an alternative method for treating diabetic polyneuropathy, although the benefits of this procedure are still controversial.[84]

**Treatment of autonomic diabetic neuropathy:** Treatments for autonomic diabetic neuropathy include improved glycemic control as some aspects (neuropathy, gastric function) may improve. Smaller, more frequent meals that are easier to digest (liquid) and low in fat and fiber may minimize symptoms of gastroparesis. A variety of agents including dopamine agonists (metoclopramide [Reglan®], 5 to 10 mg, and domperidone [Motillium™], 10 to 20 mg, before each meal) and bethanechol [Urecholine®] (10 to 20 mg before each meal) have shown some efficacy. Erythromycin (3 mg/kg/8 hours) interacts with the motilin receptor and has shown significant improvement in gastric emptying. Diabetic diarrhea in the absence of bacterial overgrowth is treated symptomatically with loperamide (Imodium®), clonidine (Catapres®) (0.6 mg three times daily) or octreotide (Sandostatin®) (50 to 75 µg three times daily subcutaneously). Treatment of bacterial overgrowth with antibiotics (metronidazole [Flagyl®]) is sometimes useful.

Patients who do not respond to the above-mentioned measures may require a botulinum toxin type A injection (Botox®) or botulinum toxin type B (Myobloc®) injection in pylorus or surgical intervention, ie, gastrostomy tube.

Therapy of orthostatic hypotension is challenging. Nonpharmacologic maneuvers (adequate sodium intake, avoidance of dehydration, and lower extremity support hose) may offer some benefit. Current pharmacologic options (clonidine, fludrocortisone, midodrine [Orvaten®, Proamatine®], and yohimbine) have had variable success but each has significant side effects.

Diabetic cystopathy should be treated with timed voiding or self-catherization. Medications like doxazosin and bethanecol may give temporary relief. The drugs for ED are sildenafil (Viagra®), tadalafil (Cialis®), and vardenafil (Levitra®), which have lower efficacy in diabetic individuals than in the nondiabetic population. Use of alprostodil and a penile implant are other options. Sexual dysfunction in women may be improved with use of vaginal lubricants, treatment of vaginal infections, and systemic or local estrogen replacement.

## Erectile Dysfunction

ED is the inability to satisfactorily achieve or maintain penile erection for sexual activity. ED is highly prevalent in diabetic men[85] and is almost always organic in its etiology. Prevalence estimates of ED in cross-sectional studies of diabetic populations range from 20% to 71%.[86] The majority of epidemiologic ED studies do not distinguish between type 1 and type 2 diabetes.

### Pathophysiology of Erectile Dysfunction in Diabetes

Normal erections are mediated by an increase in parasympathetic tone and a reduction in sympathetic tone.[87] These neural pathways are modulated by visual, auditory, olfactory, tactile, and psychological stimuli.[88] Nonadrenergic, noncholinergic nerve endings release nitric oxide (NO), which stimulates cyclic guanosine monophosphate (cGMP) in the smooth muscle of arterioles supplying the corpora cavernosa and of smooth muscle cells lining the sinusoids of the corpora cavernosa. cGMP activation initiates a fall of intracellular calcium levels, resulting in smooth muscle relaxation. The combination of increased blood flow to and the engorgement of the corpora cavernosa causes compression of the veins that drain the corpora cavernosa against the inelastic tunica albuginea. This essentially prevents venous drainage of the corpora and causes penile rigidity.

Penile tissue from diabetic men with ED demonstrates impaired neurogenic and endothelium-mediated relaxation of smooth muscle,[89] increased accumulation of AGEs,[90] and up-regulation arginase, a competitor with NO synthase for its substrate L-arginine.[91] The normal response to direct smooth muscle relaxants in most studies implies that the impairments are due to decreased synthesis, release, or activity of NO. The fundamental mechanisms mediating these changes are thought to be the same as for other diabetic complications: increased polyol pathway flux, intracellular accumulation of AGEs, activation of protein kinase C, and increased flux through the hexosamine pathway.[92]

The etiology of ED in diabetes is often multifactorial. It can result from peripheral or autonomic neuropathy (eg, nerve damage), impaired blood flow (eg, vasculopathy), nephropathy, or psychological factors. Modifiable risk factors include poor glycemic control, hypertension, increased BMI, and smoking.

### Evaluation of Erectile Dysfunction in Diabetes

Many patients with diabetes do not volunteer information about their sexual function and believe that their ED is 'in their heads' and that their physician will disregard any sexual problems they might want to discuss. Therefore, physicians should take the initiative in asking their patients sexual health.

If ED is detected, before labeling diabetes as the underlying cause, the physician should conduct a comprehensive history and physical examination to identify other possible causes of ED, such as medications, substance abuse, alcohol, hypogonadism, thyroid dysfunction, pelvic trauma, Peyronie's disease, or psychogenic causes.

The laboratory work-up should include a complete blood count (CBC), screening chemistries to rule out systemic disease, lipid profile, $HbA_{1c}$, total testosterone, leutinizing hormone (LH) level, and thyroid-stimulating hormone (TSH) level. If the total testosterone is <300 ng/dL, a second specimen should be obtained between 7 AM and 10 AM, and total testosterone, LH and prolactin should be determined. Measurement of bioavailable or free testosterone by equilibrium dialysis should be considered for borderline values or when there is reason to believe that the sex hormone-binding globulin (SHBG) level may be altered.

Depression is particularly common in diabetics, and it can be an important factor in the development of ED. It is important to differentiate psychogenic from organic ED because therapeutic interventions differ.

## Treatment of Erectile Dysfunction in Diabetes

Interestingly, no studies have demonstrated that tight glycemic control improves ED in diabetic men. However, in addition to other potential benefits, tight glycemic control can improve endothelial dysfunction, which in the early stages, may be the primary cause of ED.

### Phosphodiesterase Type 5 Inhibitors

Oral phosphodiesterase type 5 (PDE-5) inhibitors are the most prescribed drugs to treat ED. There are three FDA-approved oral agents for the treatment of ED: sildenafil, tadalafil, and vardenafil. All three PDE-5 inhibitors work by potentiating the effect of NO in the penis. They block the hydrolysis of cGMP to guanosine 5'-monophosphate, thus enhancing NO-mediated smooth muscle relaxation, increasing blood flow to the penis and facilitating erection.

There are no studies directly comparing the effectiveness of these three agents among diabetic men with ED. However, there are studies comparing the individual agents with placebo in men with type 2 diabetes and ED that demonstrate improved ability to both achieve and maintain an erection adequate for sexual intercourse with treatment.[93]

When counseling diabetic men who are considering a PDE-5 inhibitor for ED, it is important to establish realistic expectations and explain that studies have documented that all three agents are less effective in diabetic patients than in the general population of men with ED.[94,95] Patient selection for use of these agents should be conducted carefully in light of side effects. Particular caution is warranted in patients with symptomatic heart disease, as the use of these agents may precipitate an acute episode of chest pain.

## Vacuum Erection Devices

There are fragmented data available regarding the effectiveness of vacuum erection devices (VEDs) when used by diabetic men with ED. In a single-center study of 44 men with diabetes who chose a VED for the treatment of ED in the early 1990s, 75% reported that they were able to achieve erections satisfactory for intercourse with the use of the device.[96] However, there are some concerns about biased patient selection in this study. A recent review of the use of VEDs in the general treatment of ED reports low satisfaction rates with this therapy, varying between 20% and 50%.[97]

## Intraurethral Suppositories

There are no studies specifically assessing the effectiveness of prostaglandin $E_1$ ($PGE_1$) intraurethral suppositories in diabetic men. A single randomized clinical trial of the effectiveness of this agent in the general population of men with ED documented that 60% of those who tried this agent were able to achieve successful sexual intercourse.[98] Unfortunately, in clinical practice, this agent appears to be considerably less effective.

## Intracavernosal Injection Therapy

Intracavernosal (IC) injection of vasoactive agents, such as $PGE_1$, has consistently been shown to be effective in the treatment of ED in men with diabetes. In a study of 336 men with diabetes-related ED, 83% of patients reported erections satisfactory for intercourse after IC injection therapy of $PGE_1$.[99] Unfortunately, 24% of these patients also reported penile pain, one of the most common side effects of IC injection therapy. Although a considerable number of patients report penile pain with IC injection therapy, it appears that diabetic men still have high compliance rates with this therapy.

## Penile Implantation Surgery

In diabetic patients who fail medical management of ED, penile implantation surgery is a viable therapeutic option. In a recent review of 372 men who underwent implantation of a three-piece inflatable penile implant, 86% reported that the device was still functional 5 years after implantation, and 79% reported that they used the device at least twice a month.[99] There is no increased risk of infection following this procedure in diabetic men compared with nondiabetics.[100,101]

There are numerous effective therapies available for the treatment of ED in patients with diabetes. Physicians should specifically inquire about erectile function when treating their diabetic male patients and offer treatment as needed.

## References

1.    American Association of Diabetes: *All About Diabetes*. Available at: http://www.diabetes.org/about-diabetes.jsp. Accessed August 10, 2007.

2.    Prevent Blindness America 2007 website. Available at: http://www.preventblindness.org. Accessed October 19, 2007.

3.    Klein, R, Klein, BE: Vision disorders in diabetes. In: *Diabetes in America* (DHHS publication number 85-1468). Washington, DC, United States Government Printing Office, 1985, pp 293-338.

4.     Murtha T, Cavallerano J: The management of diabetic eye disease in the setting of cataract surgery. *Curr Opin Ophthalmol* 2007; 18:13-18.

5.     Writing Committee for the Diabetic Retinopathy Clinical Research Network, et al: Comparison of the modified Early Treatment Diabetic Retinopathy Study and mild macular grid laser photocoagulation strategies for diabetic macular edema. *Arch Ophthalmol* 2007;125:469-480.

6.     Cunha-Vaz J, Bernardes R: Nonproliferative retinopathy in diabetes type 2. Initial stages and characterization of phenotypes. *Prog Retin Eye Res* 2005;24:355-377.

7.     Girach A, Lund-Anderson H: Diabetic macular edema: a clinical overview. *Int J Clin Pract* 2007;61:88-97.

8.     Javitt JC, Canner JK, Frank RG, et al: Detecting and treating retinopathy in patients with type I diabetes mellitus. A health policy model. *Ophthalmology* 1997;97:483-494.

9.     Javitt JC, Aiello LP, Chiang Y, et al: Preventive eye care in people with diabetes is cost-saving to the federal government. Implications for health-care reform. *Diabetes Care* 1994;17:909-917.

10.    Klein R, Klein BEK, Moss SE, et al: The Wisconsin Epidemiologic Study of Diabetic Retinopathy. II. Prevalence and risk of diabetic retinopathy when age at diagnosis is less than 30 years. *Arch Ophthalmol* 1984;102:520-526.

11.    Early worsening of diabetic retinopathy in the Diabetes Control and Complications Trial. *Arch Ophthalmol* 1998;116:874-886.

12.    Intensive blood-glucose control with sulphonylureas or insulin compared with conventional treatment and risk of complications in patients with type 2 diabetes (UKPDS 33). UK Prospective Diabetes Study (UKPDS) Group. *Lance*t 1998;352:837-853.

13.    Ramsay RC, Goetz FC, Sutherland DE, et al: Progression of diabetic retinopathy after pancreas transplantation for insulin-dependent diabetes mellitus. *N Engl J Med* 1988;318:208-214.

14.    Tight blood pressure control and risk of macrovascular and microvascular complications in type 2 diabetes: UKPDS 38. UK Prospective Diabetes Study (UKPDS) Group. *BMJ* 1998;317:703-713.

15.    Aiello LP, Cahill MT, Wong JS: Systemic considerations in the management of diabetic retinopathy. *Am J Opthalmol* 2001; 132:760-776.

10

16.   Fong DS, Segal PP, Myers F, et al: Subretinal fibrosis in diabetic macular edema. ETDRS report number 23. Early Treatment Diabetic Retinopathy Study Research Group. *Arch Ophthalmol* 1997; 115:873-877.

17.   Klein BE, Moss SE, Klein R, et al: The Wisconsin Epidemiologic Study of Diabetic Retinopathy. XIII. Relationship of serum cholesterol to retinopathy and hard exudate. *Ophthalmology* 1991;98:1261-1265.

18.   Davis MD, Fisher MR, Gangnon RE, et al: Risk factors for high-risk proliferative diabetic retinopathy and severe vision loss: Early Treatment Diabetic Retinopathy Study Report #18. *Invest Ophthalmol Vis Sci* 1998;l39:233-252.

19.   Parving HH, Gall MA, Skott P, et al: Prevalence and causes of albuminuria in non-insulin dependent diabetic patients. *Kidney Int* 1992;41:758-762.

20.   Rosenn B, Miodovnik M, Kranias G, et al: Progression of diabetic retinopathy in pregnancy: Association with hypertension in pregnancy. *Am J Obstet Gynecol* 1992;166:1214-1218.

21.   Effects of aspirin treatment on diabetic retinopathy. ETDRS report number 8. Early Treatment Diabetic Retinopathy Study Research Group. *Ophthalmology* 1991;98(5 suppl):757-765.

22.   Effect of aspirin alone and aspirin plus dipyridamole in early diabetic retinopathy. A multicenter randomized controlled clinical trial. The DAMAD Study Group. *Diabetes* 1989;38:491-498.

23.   Ferris FL 3rd, Davis MD, Aiello LM: Treatment of diabetic retinopathy. *N Engl J Med* 1999;341:667-678.

24.   Photocoagulation treatment of proliferative diabetic retinopathy: clinical application of Diabetic Retinopathy Study (DRS) findings, DRS report number 8. Diabetic Retinopathy Study Research Group. *Ophthalmology* 1981;88:583-600.

25.   Shinoda K, Ishida S, Kawashima S, et al: Clinical factors related to the aqueous levels of vascular endothelial growth factor and hepatocyte growth factor in progressive diabetic retinopathy. *Curr Eye Res* 2000;21:655-661.

26.   Stefansson E, Machemer R, De Juan E Jr, et al: Retinal oxygenation and laser treatment in patients with diabetic retinopathy. *Am J Ophthalmol* 1992;113:36-38.

27.   Early vitrectomy for severe vitreous hemorrhage in diabetic retinopathy. Two-year results of a randomized trial. Diabetic Retinopathy

Vitrectomy Study Report 2. The Diabetic Retinopathy Vitrectomy Study Research Group. *Arch Ophthalmol* 1985;103:1644-1652.

28. Renal Data System, USRDS 2007 annual data report. Bethesda, MD, National Institute of Diabetes and Digestive and Kidney Diseases, 2007. Available at: http://www.usrds.org/adr.htm. Accessed October 19, 2007.

29. Trevisan R, Viberti G: Genetic factors in the development of diabetic nephropathy. *J Lab Clin Med* 1995;126:342-349.

30. Brancati FL, Whittle JC, Whelton PK, et al: The excess incidence of diabetic end-stage renal disease among blacks. A population-based study of potential explanatory factors. *JAMA* 1992;268:3079-3084.

31. Tapp RJ, Shaw JE, Zimmet PZ, et al: Albuminuria is evident in the early stages of diabetes onset: results from the Australian Diabetes, Obesity, and Lifestyle Study (AusDiab). *Am J Kidney Dis* 2004;44:792-798.

32. Parving HH, Hommel E, Mathiesen E, et al: Prevalence of microalbuminuria, arterial hypertension, retinopathy and neuropathy in patients with insulin dependent diabetes. *Br Med J Clin Res Ed* 1988;296:156-160.

33. Ritz E, Orth SR: Nephropathy in patients with type 2 diabetes mellitus. *N Engl J Med* 1999;341:1127-1133.

34. Jermendy G, Ruggenenti P: Preventing microalbuminuria in patients with type 2 diabetes. *Diabetes Metab Res Rev* 2007;23:100-110.

35. Levine DZ: Hyperfiltration, nitric oxide, and diabetic nephropathy. *Curr Hypertens Rep* 2006;8:153-157.

36. Toyoda M, Suzuki D, Honma M, et al: High expression of PKC-MAPK pathway mRNAs correlates with glomerular lesions in human diabetic nephropathy. *Kidney Int* 2004;66:1107-14.

37. Gandjour A, Lauterbach KW: An evidence based disease management program for patients with diabetic nephropathy. *J Nephrol* 2003;16:500-510.

38. Friedman EA, Friedman AL, Eggers P: End-stage renal disease in diabetic persons: is the pandemic subsiding? *Kidney Int* 2006;104(suppl):S51-S54.

39. Standards of Medical Care in Diabetes Recommendations 2007: *Diabetes Care* 2007;30(suppl 1):S4-S41.

10

40.   Mogensen CE, Vestbo E, Poulsen PL, et al: Microalbuminuria and potential confounders. A review and some observations on variability of urinary albumin excretion. *Diabetes Care* 1995;18:572-581.

41.   The effect of intensive treatment of diabetes on the development and progression of long-term complications in insulin-dependent diabetes mellitus. The Diabetes Control and Complications Trial Research Group. *N Engl J Med* 1993;329:977-986.

42.   Writing Team for Diabetes Control and Complications Trial/ Epidemiology of Diabetic Interventions and Complications Research Group: Effect of intensive therapy on the microvascular complications of type 1 diabetes mellitus. *JAMA* 2002;287:2563-2569.

43.   Meloni C, Tatangelo P, Cipriani S, et al: Adequate dietary restriction in diabetic and nondiabetic patients with chronic renal failure. *J Ren Nutr* 2004;14:208-213.

44.   Sengul AM, Altuntas Y, Kurklu A, et al: Beneficial effect of lisinopril plus telmisartan in patients with type 2 diabetes, microalbuminuria, and hypertension. *Diabetes Res Clin Pract* 2006;71: 210-219.

45.   Lewis EJ, Hunsicker LG, Bain RP, et al: The effect of angiotensin concerting enzyme inhibition on diabetic nephropathy. The Collaborative Study Group. *N Engl J Med* 1993;329:1456-1462.

46.   Adler AI, Stratton IM, Neil HA, et al: Association of systolic blood pressure with macrovascular and microvascular complications of type 2 diabetes (UKPDS 36): prospective observational study. *BMJ* 2000;321:412-419.

47.   ALLHAT Officers and Coordinators for ALLHAT Collaborative Research Group. The Antihypertensive and Lipid-Lowering Treatment to Prevent Heart Attack Trial: Major outcomes in high-risk hypertensive patients randomized to angiotensin-converting enzyme inhibitor or calcium channel blocker vs diuretic: The Antihypertensive and Lipid-Lowering Treatment to Prevent Heart Attack Trial (ALLHAT). *JAMA* 2002;288:2981-2997.

48.   Gerstein HC: Reduction of cardiovascular events and microvascular complications in diabetes with ACE inhibitor treatment: HOPE and MICRO-HOPE. *Diabetes Metab Res Rev* 2002;18(suppl 3): S82-S85.

49.   Brenner BM, Cooper ME, de Zeeuw D, et al: Effects of losartan on renal and cardiovascular outcomes in patients with type 2 diabetes and nephropathy. *N Engl J Med* 2001;345:861-869.

50. Brenner BM, Cooper ME, de Zeeuw D, et al: The losartan renal protection study— rationale, study design and baseline characteristics of RENAAL (Reduction of Endpoints in NIDDM with the Angiotensin II Antagonist Losartan). *J Renin Angiotensin Aldosterone Syst* 2000;1:328-335.

51. Mogensen CE, Neldam S, Tikkanen I, et al: Randomised controlled trial of dual blockade of renin-angiotensin system in patients with hypertension, microalbuminuria, and non-insulin dependent diabetes: the candesartan and lisinopril microalbuminuria (CALM) study. *BMJ* 2000;321:1440-1444.

52. Han SY, Kim CH, Kim HS, et al: Spironolactone prevents diabetic nephropathy through an anti-inflammatory mechanism in type 2 diabetic rats. *J Am Soc Nephrol* 2006;17:1362-1372.

53. Nielsen FS, Rossing P, Gall MA, et al: Impact of lisinopril and atenolol on kidney function in hypertensive NIDDM subjects with diabetic nephropathy. *Diabetes* 1994;43:1108-1113.

54. Bakris GL, Barnhill BW, Sadler R: Treatment of arterial hypertension in diabetic humans: importance of therapeutic selection. *Kidney Int* 1992;41:912-919.

55. Rosenberger J, van Dijk JP, Nagyova I, et al: Do dialysis- and transplantation-realted medical factors affect perceived health status? *Nephrol Dial Transplant* 2005;20:2153-2158.

56. Fiorina P, Venturini M, Folli F, et al: Natural history of kidney graft survival, hypertrophy, and vascular function in end-stage renal disease type 1 diabetic kidney-transplanted patients:beneficial impact of pancreas and successful islet cotransplantation. *Diabetes Care* 2005;28:1303-1310.

57. Boulton AJ, Gries FA, Jervell JA: Guidelines for the diagnosis and outpatient management of diabetic peripheral neuropathy. *Diabet Med* 1998;15:508-514.

58. Spruce MC, Potter J, Coppini DV: The pathogenesis and management of painful diabetic neuropathy. *Diabet Med* 2003;20: 88-98.

59. Thomas PK: Classification of the diabetic neuropathies. In: Gries FA, Cameron NE, Low PA, et al, eds: *Textbook of Diabetic Neuropathy.* Stuttgart, Germany, Thieme, 2003, pp 175-177.

60. Boulton AJM, Malik RA: Diabetic neuropathy. *Med Clin N Am* 1998;82:909-929.

10

61. Jude EB, Boulton AJM: End-stage complications of diabetic neuropathy. *Diabetes Rev* 1999;7:395-410.

62. Vinik AI, Ziegler D: Diabetic cardiovascular autonomic neuropathy. *Circulation* 2007;115:387-397.

63. Vinik AI, Erbas T: Cardiovascular autonomic neuropathy: diagnosis and management. *Curr Diab Rep* 2006;6:424-430.

64. The definition of orthostatic hypotension, pure autonomic failure, and multiple system atrophy. *J Auton Nerv Syst* 1996;58:123-124.

65. Prevalence of unrecognized silent ischemia and its association with atherosclerotic risk factors in noninsulin-dependent diabetes mellitus. Milan Study on Athersclerosis and Diabetes (MiSAD) Group. *Am J Cardiol* 1997;79:134-139.

66. Bytzer P, Talley NJ, Leemon M, et al: Prevalence of gastrointestinal symptoms associated with diabetes mellitus: a population-based survey of 15,000 adults. *Arch Intern Med* 2001;161:1989-1996.

67. Maxton DG, Whorwell PJ: Functional bowel symptoms in diabetes—the role of autonomic neuropathy. *Postgrad Med J* 1991; 67:991-993.

68. Brown JS, Wessells H, Chancellor MB, et al: Urologic complications of diabetes. *Diabetes Care* 2005;28:177-185.

69. Ellenburg M: Development of urinary bladder dysfunction in diabetes mellitus. *Ann Intern Med* 1980;92:321-323.

70. Norden G, Granerus G, Nybetg G: Diabetic cystopathy—a risk factor in diabetic neprhropathy? *J Diabet Complications* 1988;2: 203-206.

71. Bacon CG, Hu FB, Rimm EB: Association of type and duration of diabetes with erectile dysfunction in a large cohort of men. *Diabetes Care* 2002;25:1458-1463.

72. Vinik AI, Richradson D: Erectile dysfunction in diabetes. *Diabetes Rev* 1998;6:16-33.

73. Enzlin P, Mathieu C, Demyttenaere K: Diabetes mellitus and female sexuality: a review of 25 years' research. *Diabet Med* 1998;15: 809-815.

74. Fealey RD, Low PA, Thomas JE: Thermoregulatory sweating abnormalities in diabetes mellitus. *Mayo Clin Proc* 1989;64:617-628.

75. Meyer C, Grossmann R, Mitrakou A, et al: Effects of autonomic neuropathy on counterregulation and awareness of hypoglycemia in type 1 diabetic patients. *Diabetes Care* 1998;21:1960-1966.

76.  Boulton JM, Malik AR, Sosenko JM: Diabetic Somatic Neuropathies. *Diabetes Care* 2004;27:1458-1486.

77.  Richards BW, Jones FR, Young BR: Causes and prognosis in 4,278 cases of paralysis of oculomotor, trochlear, and abducens cranial nerves. *Am J Ophthalmol* 1992;113:489-496.

78.  Abrahim-Inpijn L, Oosting J, Hart AA: Bell's palsy: Factors affecting prognosis in 200 patients with reference to hypertension and diabetes mellitus. *Clin Otolaryngol* 1987;12:349-355.

79.  Stevens JC, Smith BE: Cranial reflexes. In: Daube JR, ed: *Clinical Neurophysiology*. Philadelphia, PA, FA Davis, 1996, pp 321-335.

80.  Katz JN, Larson MG, Sabra A, et al: The carpal tunnel syndrome: diagnostic utility of the history and physical examination findings. *Ann Intern Med* 1990:112:321-327.

81.  Dyck PJ, Windebank AJ: Diabetic and nondiabetic lumbosacral radicloplexus neuropathies: new insight into pathophysiology and treatment. *Muscle Nerve* 2002;25:477-491.

82.  Haq RU, Pendlebury WW, Fries TJ, et al: Chronic inflammatory demyelinating polyradiculopathy in diabetic patients. *Muscle Nerve* 2003;27:465-470.

83.  Kumar D, Marshall HJ: Diabetic peripheral neuropathy: amelioration of pain with transcutaneous electrostimulation. *Diabetes Care* 1997;20:1702-1705.

84.  Dellon AL: Treatment of symptomatic diabetic neuropathy by surgical decompression of multiple peripheral nerves. *Plast Reconstr Surg* 1992;89:689-697.

85.  Klein R, Klein BE, Lee KE, et al: Prevalence of self-reported erectile dysfunction in people with long-term IDDM. *Diabetes Care* 1996;19:135-141.

86.  Penson DF, Wessells H: Erectile dysfunction in diabetic patients. *Diabetes Spectrum* 2004;17:225-230.

87.  Andersson KE, Wagner G: Physiology of penile erection. *Physiol Rev* 1995;75:191-236.

88.  Lue TF: Erectile dysfunction. *N Engl J Med* 2000;342:1802-1813.

89.  Saenz de Tejada I, Goldstein I, Azadzoi K, et al: Impaired neurogenic and endothelium-mediated relaxation of penile smooth

10

muscle from diabetic men with impotence. *N Engl J Med* 1989;320: 1025-1030.

90.  Seftel AD, Vaziri ND, Ni Z, et al: Advanced glycation end products in human penis: elevation in diabetic tissue, site of deposition, and possible effect through iNOS or eNOS. *Urology* 1997;50: 1016-1026.

91.  Bivalacqua TJ, Hellstrom WJ, Kadowitz PJ, et al: Increased expression of arginase II in human diabetic corpus cavernosum: in diabetic-associated erectile dysfunction. *Biochem Biophys Res Commun* 2001,283:923-927.

92.  Brownlee M: Biochemistry and molecular cell biology of diabetic complications. *Nature* 2001;414:813-820.

93.  Boulton AJ, Selam JL, Sweeney M, et al: Sildenafil citrate for the treatment of erectile dysfunction in men with type II diabetes mellitus. *Diabetologia* 2001;44:1296-1301.

94.  Carson CC 3rd: Sildenafil: a 4-year update in the treatment of 20 million erectile dysfunction patients. *Curr Urol Rep* 2003;4: 488-496.

95.  Jarow JP, Burnett AL, Geringer AM: Clinical efficacy of sildenafil citrate based on etiology and response to prior treatment. *J Urol* 1999;162:722-725.

96.  Price DE, Cooksey G, Jehu D, et al: The management of impotence in diabetic men by vacuum tumescence therapy. *Diabet Med* 1991;8:964-967.

97.  Levine LA, Dimitriou RJ: Vacuum constriction and external erection devices in erectile dysfunction. *Urol Clin North Am* 2001;28:335-341.

98.  Padma-Nathan H, Hellstrom WJ, Tam PY, et al: Treatment of men with erectile dysfunction with transurethral alprostadil. *N Engl J Med* 1997;336:1-7.

99.  Heaton JP, Lording D, Liu SN, et al: Intracavernosal alprostadil is effective for the treatment of erectile dysfunction in diabetic men. *Int J Impot Res* 2001,13:317-321.

100. Carson CC, Mulcahy JJ, Govier FE: Efficacy, safety and patient satisfaction outcomes of the AMS 700CX inflatable penile prosthesis: results of a long-term multicenter study. *J Urol* 2000;164:376-380.

101. Lotan Y, Roehrborn CG, McConnell JD, et al: Factors influencing the outcomes of penile prosthesis surgery at a teaching institution. *Urology* 2003;62:918-921.

# Index

# NOTES

# Contemporary Diagnosis and Management of The Patient With Type 2 Diabetes®

Retail $19.95

## Ordering Information

### Prices (in U.S. dollars)

| | |
|---|---|
| 1 book: | $19.95 each |
| 2-9 books: | $17.96 each |
| 10-99 books: | $15.96 each |
| > 99 books: | Call 800-860-9544* |

### How to Order:

1. by telephone: 800-860-9544*
2. by fax: 215-860-9558
3. by Internet: www.HHCbooks.com
4. by mail: Handbooks in Health Care Co.
    3 Terry Drive, Suite 201
    Newtown, PA 18940

### Shipping/Handling

**Books will be shipped via or UPS or DHL Ground unless otherwise requested.**

| | |
|---|---|
| 1-3 books: | $6.00 |
| 4-9 books: | $8.00 |
| 10-14 books: | $11.00 |
| 15-24 books: | $13.00 |
| > 24 books: | Plus shipping |

International orders: Please inquire

*Please call between 9 AM and 5 PM EST Monday through Friday, 800-860-9544.

Pennsylvania residents must add 6% sales tax.

*Prices good through December 31, 2008*